55
126, PIC
148        166
        162

# GO FROM
# STRESSED TO
# STRONG

# GO FROM
# STRESSED TO STRONG

## Health and Fitness Advice from High Achievers

### LAURIE A. WATKINS

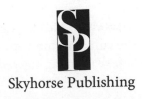

Skyhorse Publishing

Skyhorse Publishing books may be purchased in bulk at special discounts for sales promotion, corporate gifts, fund-raising, or educational purposes. Special editions can also be created to specifications. For details, contact the Special Sales Department, Skyhorse Publishing, 307 West 36th Street, 11th Floor, New York, NY 10018 or info@skyhorsepublishing.com.

Skyhorse® and Skyhorse Publishing® are registered trademarks of Skyhorse Publishing, Inc.®, a Delaware corporation.

Visit our website at www.skyhorsepublishing.com.

10 9 8 7 6 5 4 3 2 1

Library of Congress Cataloging-in-Publication Data is available on file.

Cover design by Chelsey Marie
Cover photo credit Laura Metzler

ISBN: 978-1-5107-1653-7
Ebook ISBN: 978-1-5107-1654-4
Printed in the United States of America

**Disclaimer**
**This book presents the research and ideas of its author. It is not intended to replace the consultation with a professional healthcare practitioner before starting any reset, diet, or supplement regimen.**

To all those who continue to put everything and everyone else before themselves; this book was written for you. May you live consciously and deliberately, never allowing anyone or anything to come in between your ultimate health and happiness—even yourself.

# CONTENTS

CHAPTER 1: FEELING THE BURNOUT?                                    1

CHAPTER 2: GET OUT OF BED AND FALL INTO A ROUTINE                 17

CHAPTER 3: HIGH-SPEED FUEL                                        42

CHAPTER 4: SLEEP IS NOT FOR THE WEAK                              85

CHAPTER 5: CHILL OUT AND TAKE A MOMENT TO BREATHE               106

CHAPTER 6: PROTECT YOUR WORKOUT BY MAKING IT
           A PRIORITY                                            137

CHAPTER 7: TIME MANAGEMENT                                       157

CHAPTER 8: THE HOME STRETCH                                      176


APPENDIX                                                         190

ACKNOWLEDGMENTS                                                  205

ENDNOTES                                                         209

# CHAPTER 1

# FEELING THE BURNOUT?

E ver wonder what's the scariest thing about burnout? Here's the cold hard truth: you won't even see it coming, because it usually happens when you're doing something that you're passionate about, and quite good at.

Burnout is not some made-up thing lazy people pretend to have (like a cold) so they can stay home, avoiding the office. It's a force stronger than a hurricane that can knock you out completely, making even the simplest of tasks like getting dressed and showered, cooking a meal, or answering email seem impossible. You don't get burned out because you're weak. You get burned out because you've tried to stay strong for far too long.

I assume you must have felt, or dare I say currently feel, as though "total destruction" were nipping at your heels or you wouldn't have picked up this book looking for help. By now I hope you recognize that at some point you've more than likely enabled yourself to play the supporting role in the movie of your own life. Seriously, think about that for a second. We have all allowed someone or something to dictate our time and misalign our priorities, at the expense of our own health and well-being. I've been there a few times; hell, I've been there more than a few times. Who am I kidding?

It was 9:07 p.m., I was driving on Alligator Alley across the good 'ole Sunshine State, and Caroline Kennedy was waiting. The temperature through the Everglades was still a blistering 80 degrees, even though it was late October. It was the last week of the 2008 presidential campaign, and Kennedy would be stumping for then-Senator Barack Obama the following morning. Stumping is a crucial part of campaigning, and an opportunity for potential voters to meet candidates and their surrogates. Stump speeches are usually designed to be used in several locations within a state, conveying the same basic ideas at each stop. Staff members will rework the speech slightly for each location, subtly changing the focus depending on the audience. In this case, it was my job to bring Kennedy up to speed on the key political and policy issues in the state of Florida and travel with her across the state over the next few days.

Suddenly, a sharp pain punched me in the gut. I slouched over, briefly taking my eyes off the road. I rubbed my stomach gingerly as I forced myself to focus on the road and searched for a clue as to what was causing the pain. Then it hit me: the only thing I had eaten all day was a cinnamon and brown sugar Pop-Tart, over nine hours before. I don't think any nutritionist would have given me extra credit for the seven cups of coffee I had pumped into my body either, hoping it would fuel me through the rest of my long day.

But after all, this was presidential campaigning; meals were for the weak, right? I remember the first piece of advice I ever received while working on my first campaign right out of college: "Eat when you can." After only a brief period of time working on the campaign, I knew the game and thought I knew how to play it pretty well. Yet, this time I felt faint, and the pain would not go away. That was the moment I realized I was out of control, had a problem, and needed to make a change.

A political campaign feels unique to those inside it, but it's very similar to any other campaign—that is, a goal-oriented activity that occurs in a finite period of time. One minute you could be sitting in a cubicle, elbows brushing against another employee, and the next you're in the back of an SUV briefing a celebrity, a CEO, or even the Vice President of the United States. The pace is invigorating, but the demands are exhausting. After seven long months, by the end of the 2008 presidential campaign, I found myself in the same place that so many others do when their work and life are out of balance—with a toxic diet, lousy sleeping habits, an irregular exercise schedule, and a sense of general physical distress. By trying to give everything I had to my work, I ended up without the energy to be of any use to myself or the campaign. And after it was over, I was left with nothing but "hope and change," gray hair, and twelve extra pounds. By the last week of the campaign, I had hit the lowest point possible—I had to change.

The long hours, lightning-speed pace, and demand of the job as political director eventually took its toll on my health. I made small changes, which brought temporary relief, but the problems only followed me to Washington, DC, and to my next job at the Pentagon. Falling into the same unhealthy patterns as I did on the campaign and fearing disaster, I made the decision to take control of my life.

In 2010, I joined a CrossFit gym, changed my diet and sleeping habits, and learned how to efficiently manage my time and stress even while working in a high-performing job. In 2012, I moved back to Florida to work on President Obama's reelection campaign as his policy director. Fearful that all the hard work and progress I made with my health and fitness since the last campaign would be destroyed by the horrendous and unsustainable schedule, I developed my own program. With a mastery in 5 areas—time management, sleep, food, fitness, and stress management—this program allowed me to align my professional and personal life, finding my own strength in the face of adversity.

I have a strong belief that it isn't just about being able to get through difficult "campaigns" throughout your life, but it's also about preparing yourself—both physically and mentally—for the tests that life will put you through. In this book, I will provide you with practical and proven tools I designed based on the advice of health and wellness experts to get you on the path to a healthy lifestyle in a 24-7 world. Prompted by my own experiences while working inside the world of two presidential campaigns, the Pentagon, Capitol Hill, and other stress-filled environments, I will share my own anecdotes as well as stories from prominent men and women across a wide range of industries on their experiences and how they survived that particular "campaign" in their life and came out the other side. Strong.

While my story plays out on the political stage, I designed this book for anyone with a busy lifestyle who thinks he or she can't fit in being healthy. Whether you're a CEO, a full-time student, a CPA during tax season, an entrepreneur, or a full-time parent—with a little hard work and determination, you can achieve your best self simply by making a few changes and sticking to them. As the pace of life continues to accelerate and the stress of our daily routine presses on every free moment, many of us put off being healthy for another day. "I'll lose the weight after the campaign," we said as we stuffed ourselves with free pizza. Or "as soon as the kids are older I'll get back to the gym." But seizing control and taking command of today was what gave me the energy and strength to make it through the next day, and the day after, and the day after that.

The myth of the campaign trail has spawned countless books on political campaign strategy, postmortems on their failures and triumphs, and autobiographies of every major player. But there is another story, and one that is seldom spoken about: the behind-the-scenes life of the campaigner, the staffer who works from seven a.m. to midnight, seven days a week, traveling to every event, writing every speech, running offense with the press, and ensuring that every train runs on time. What you wear, say, how you conduct yourself, and when you take a vacation is all dependent upon the schedule and priorities of the person or organization you work for. As for your life, well, it comes second, of course. More likely than not you've performed similar duties, perhaps from under a different job title.

In the following pages, you'll find my lifestyle guidance to help mitigate the destructive impact of certain choices on body, mind, and spirit, and how to thrive despite those choices. Grounded in science and informed by real-life experiences of what does and does not work, *Go from Stressed to Strong* shares my knowledge, along with the skills and know-how gained by busy people through their personal experiences and from consulting with health and nutrition experts.

As you read this book, you're going to learn

- how to feed yourself deliciously and nutritiously while on the run
- how important it is to keep moving at your own pace, and not at the pace that others set for you
- techniques of time management and how to better balance work, life, and staying healthy
- how to sleep better, steadily increasing your time under the sheets until you hit the ideal sleep time for you.

If you take away nothing else from this book, I hope you will gain the understanding that *nutrition, fitness, awareness,* and *discipline* are not just words; they are tools. They are power. They are ways to take care of yourself even in the harshest of working environments, tools to empower you to be stronger, smarter, happier, and truer to yourself.

I'm not a scientist or doctor. My expertise is strategies and tactics that build competitive organizations. I'm now an entrepreneur, and a woman who has spent the last fourteen years of her career learning about what my body and mind are capable of when cared for properly. And it was only when I was stretched too thin and had burned the candle at both ends that I decided I needed a change. Because I want you to be able to thrive in your personal and professional lives and avoid burnout, I spoke to people who at some point in their life have also been through similarly grueling campaigns and share their knowledge with you throughout the book. I found that even the most successful people around the world have dealt with this challenge at some point, and it's what they did to reset and recover that changed their life and career forever.

Meet my **"Strength Seekers."** They include:

**Bill Nye the Science Guy** quit his engineering job and decided to become a performer after growing tired of working for people predominantly focused on the bottom line, sometimes at the expense of others. In 2013, Bill landed a spot on the TV show *Dancing with the Stars* and started to train, working his upper body. Yet shortly into the season, he tore his quadriceps tendon during a taped rehearsal, in front of millions of viewers. During his initial evaluation, Bill asked, "how did this happen?" to which the sports medicine doctor replied, "Well, you're old." That was all Bill needed to hear to really kick-start his workout regimen, changing everything about his overall health and well-being.

**José Andrés** is a two-star Michelin-awarded chef, restaurateur, and humanitarian who admits that "kitchens have always been a stressful place" and was once on the receiving end of a "pan-throwing" chef. As a result, he vowed never to run his kitchens like that. Dedicated to exploring the possibility of what healthy, fresh food can do for the world, he went on to found Beefsteak, a revolutionary fast-casual restaurant the aim of which is to improve the way Americans eat, by putting vegetables at the core of the meal.

**Elissa Goodman**, after graduating from college, wanted the fast life of a "successful" businesswoman. She worked long hours at a stressful job, fueling herself with caffeine and expensive restaurant dinners. Exercise was a luxury, and sleep was for those who didn't care about moving up the ladder. She wanted to conquer the world. Then she felt a lump. When the doctor told her she had Hodgkin's lymphoma, she was stunned. Elissa had just gotten married and was planning to start a family. She was only thirty-two—too young to get cancer. Her doctor recommended chemotherapy and radiation, but after a few treatments she felt like the "solution" was worse than the problem. She realized that, in addition to medical treatment, her body needed nourishment and love. After a lot of research and listening to her inner voice, she shortened her radiation regimen and pursued an alternative path. She left her job, began managing her stress and doing yoga, and learned that what people had told her was good food wasn't really healthy food at all. She began juicing and eating a more plant-based diet, and within a few months she began to heal.

**Congressman Tim Ryan (OH)**, after logging thousands of miles a year, doing constant fund-raising, being away from his family, and having to endure the ever-constant environment of hyper-partisanship, as well as the stress from the job, felt himself beginning to burn out. He discovered meditation and yoga and has been able to maintain his routine while also serving as a busy member of Congress. He's responsible for bringing *Yoga on the Hill* to the U.S. Capitol in order to make yoga more accessible to members and staff and to promote mental and physical wellness. Yoga teaches patience and acceptance, qualities that make better public servants. He is also the author of *The Real Food Revolution: Healthy Eating,*

*Green Groceries, and the Return of the American Family Farm* and *A Mindful Nation: How a Simple Practice Can Help Us Reduce Stress, Improve Performance, and Recapture the American Spirit.*

**Lori Garver** led the NASA (National Aeronautics and Space Administration) transition team for the incoming Obama administration in 2008–2009 and served as NASA's deputy administrator from 2009 to 2013, all while balancing the role of mother, wife, and boss. Lori's moment came during a staff meeting at NASA while serving as the head of policy during the Clinton Administration. Overhearing that Lori, along with some of her colleagues, were planning to train for the Marine Corps Marathon, a senior official, who Lori knew was not her biggest fan, flippantly blurted out, "she could never do it." Well, that was all the motivation Lori would need to kick-start her workout routine and training.

**Dan Nevins**, professional speaker and Army veteran, shares his story of service on and off the battlefield, as well as the lessons learned as a bilateral amputee living with a traumatic brain injury (TBI). After he endured thirty-some surgeries, stayed at Walter Reed Army Medical Center for two years, and integrated back into civilian life, the invisible wounds of war started to surface. What a bike ride or golf clubs used to provide as relief before his injuries was now something of the past. The wounds became omnipresent and intrusive and prevented him from going to sleep. When his body would finally allow him to rest, he would be awoken again by nightmares. He said, "If I had to stay like that for a year or longer, I would have become one of those twenty-two service members a day who take their own life." Dan's story of how yoga profoundly changed his life continues to be his source of inspiration to lead fellow wounded warriors to yoga, mindfulness, and meditation.

**Jamie Leeds**, chef and owner of Hank's Oyster Bar, was extremely overweight, had become hobbled by arthritis, and was in so much pain that walking up the stairs or standing for long periods of time was unbearable. After more than thirty years working in kitchens and running restaurants, she was paying the price for decades of being on her feet, under pressure, and working day and night with food. She realized it was time for a drastic change, fearing her weight and pain would suppress her personal and professional growth. Jamie underwent duodenal switch (DS) surgery in 2013 and has since lost 160 pounds and kept it off—a feat that has overhauled her entire outlook on eating and what she serves in her restaurants.

**Dr. Ronald L. Kotler**, prominent sleep expert and frequent guest on *The Oprah Winfrey Show*, is a pulmonologist and respiratory director at the Pennsylvania Hospital Sleep Disorders Center and coauthor of *365 Ways to Get a Good Night's Sleep* and *20 Years Younger*. Dr. Kotler discusses how proper sleep habits and hygiene are essential to good health. He says, "Not getting enough sleep can actually shorten your life." He recommends good sleep habits and hygiene, including getting to bed at the same time every night, getting eight hours of sleep, and more.

**Christy Adkins**, one of the most respected and decorated women in the sport of CrossFit, jumped into the sport in 2007. She would go on to achieve Top 10 finishes at the CrossFit Games in 2009, 2010, and 2013 and earned the title of the twenty-fourth "Fittest Woman on Earth" in 2016. But Christy didn't always eat, sleep, or take care of herself the way she does now. Christy's moment came during the year after she graduated from college at George Washington University in DC. She had gone from living in the dorm to living with her two best friends from college just a few blocks away from their old dorm building. Christy admits she was still very much living in "party mode." Despite the fact that she had a job, followed her own training regimen, and was a personal trainer at a gym, advocating a healthy lifestyle to her clients, she was still drinking a lot and eating poorly late at night. Christy would eat pretty well for breakfast and lunch, but then by dinner, bar food, takeout, and junk became the go-tos. At the urging of her friend and trainer, she tried the Zone Diet and became conscious of incorporating one protein, a carbohydrate, and a healthy fat into each meal. This positive change in diet led to an immediate transformation of body composition, results in the gym, and improved sleep. It has shaped her overall health and wellness, making her an incredible athlete and competitor.

**Jacob "Jake" Frank**, park ranger and videographer at Yellowstone National Park, was studying to be an industrial engineer at the University of Florida. After surviving a bad motorcycle accident, he asked himself, "Is this really what I want to do with my life: sit in a cubicle?" He decided to do something spontaneous—sign up for a Parks and Recreation class, an experience that he thoroughly enjoyed and eventually prompted him to change his major. After landing an internship in the Grand Tetons, he discovered that there was an entire career built around being outside with nature. He immediately gravitated toward the happy people there who all seemed to enjoy their jobs and decided that he wanted to live and work where people wanted to go on vacation. He made the switch, never looking back.

**Stacey Colino** is a freelance Health & Wellness reporter at *U.S. News*. An award-winning writer specializing in health, fitness, psychology and nutrition, her work has appeared in dozens of national magazines, including *Prevention*, *Health*, *Newsweek*, *Women's Health*, *Parents*, *Family Circle*, and *Real Simple*. In addition, she is the coauthor of *Disease-Proof: The Remarkable Truth About What Makes Us Well* with Dr. David Katz; *Strong Is the New Skinny* with Jennifer Cohen; and *Good Food—Fast!* with Chef Jason Roberts. She is also a certified spinning and group exercise instructor. Stacey offers ideas on developing a routine, which I've broken down into a set of 20 key points in Chapter 2.

**Phil Larson**, former senior advisor for space and innovation at the White House as well as communications rainmaker at Space X for Elon Musk, and currently assistant dean for communications, strategy, and planning at the University of Colorado Boulder's College of Engineering and Applied Science, finally hit his breaking point in 2014. Phil's also my friend, and while we were both at the annual Space

Symposium in Colorado Springs, we decided to head over to nearby Garden of the Gods during some downtime for a moderate hike. Out of shape, winded, and looking to me for relief, Phil shouted, "Stop! I don't like *not* being able to breathe, even if I am in Colorado at five thousand feet." Right then and there, he proclaimed to me and to himself, "I can't do this anymore. I have to make a change." With my help and a nutrition plan of a strict Paleo diet, moderate exercise, and increased sleep, he lost thirty-five pounds. Since doing the reset, Phil has learned how to create a better work-life balance that is sustainable and manageable even while working for a company that deals in rocket science, where maintaining focus and accuracy is critical. The stress factor can be severe, like when the company launched a new satellite and something went wrong. These things cost between $150 million and $1 billion, and sometimes it comes down to that moment, trying to save a mission that took years to design and test.

**Cadet Austin Willard** enrolled in the United States Military Academy at West Point in July 2013 and is due to graduate in the Spring of 2017. The former rugby player and engineering major discusses life as a nontraditional college student in an environment where everything from the clothes he wears to the food he eats is dictated and measured. The grind is relentless, wearing people down over time. Forced to be on top of his game seven days a week and with no chance to catch his breath, Austin shares advice on what got him through his toughest challenge yet. For Austin, being fit is more about one's health and abilities than it is about simply passing the

APFT (the Academy's Physical Fitness Test)—it's a lifestyle. He takes his job very seriously and hopes to become an infantry officer upon graduation. He explains, "Fitness is a big part of being a leader in the Army. You can't lead officers if you're not in great shape yourself. Your soldiers are going to expect you to be."

In my career, I have held high-pressure, high-profile slots on two presidential campaigns, worked in Congress, served as an Obama Administration appointee assigned to the Pentagon, barely came out alive working as a defense and aerospace business development executive, and now I'm onto my most exciting role yet: author and entrepreneur. Ultimately, the stress and nonstop demands took a toll on me physically. It was only after going through the 2008 presidential campaign that I reached my limit and decided something had to give. With hard work and determination, I was able to change that into vibrant health, restful sleep, and good-for-me habits.

This book is written by one of your own. We share the perspective and attitude of today's busy professionals. We can be living proof that a healthier lifestyle makes us better leaders, colleagues, partners, family members, and friends.

With the economic market currently on the rebound, an increasing number of Americans are asking themselves how they can not only survive longer, but also live a more purpose-driven and fulfilling life. I wrote this book to help motivate people to get started in achieving a healthier life, even in the most adverse situations. You've been needing this reset for a long time, whether or not you realize it. Only you can control what your future self looks like. Do you want to look worn down, haggard, and left feeling checked out at the end of each day? I imagine that you don't.

If you want to feel happy and healthy and look bright again, then you have come to the right place. You already know how to maintain yourself; eat, shower, sleep, repeat. But what I want to teach you is how to take care of yourself. *Really* take care of yourself. Of course, it's important to take care of your basic health needs—hydrating, eating well, getting enough sleep, and physical activity. I want to take you to the next level, but you have to be ready and willing to be selfish (yes, selfish) and resourceful.

Taking care of yourself is a must. It is not separate from your work or business. By the time you finish this book, you will learn the meaning of *Work Life Integration* and *hopefully* come to live by it. You will learn new good-for-you habits that will help you set priorities for what's important and what needs to be done that day. I will share with you my program proven to help "Command Your Day Now$^{TM}$," addressing each of the five areas most people struggle to keep well aligned: nutrition, exercise, sleep, stress management, and time management.

By asking yourself each morning, "What are my business tasks?" and "What are my life tasks?" you can begin to make a list, eventually combining the two, throwing out those with the lowest priority. There are only so many hours in each day, and the way these tools will work is through effective time management. It is the pillar and foundation to living a life where you are thriving, not simply surviving. I will teach you how to be ruthless with your time, eliminating those people and things that don't serve your top five priorities. You, too, can create an amazing support system in your life by enrolling like-minded, supportive, strong people into your vision. Are there people in your life or business that aren't committed to a greater purpose and cause? If the answer is yes, then how do you expect to show up and be your best self? To get stuff done, you should surround yourself with people who do two things: 1. Cheer for you and 2. Hold you accountable.

Stress stops us from gaining momentum. Whatever setback has delayed your plan of exercising in the morning before work, remembering to eat lunch, getting more sleep, and being more present and intentional in your relationships with people at work and outside of the office, that's okay. It is time to move on. You need to be right here, right now in order to be ready to receive the necessary tools and methods that will put you on the right path toward your new life of health and happiness.

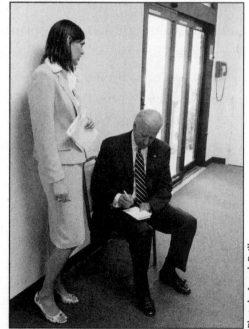

Photo by Joseph Reilly

*Laurie A. Watkins advising Vice President Joe Biden at a campaign stop in Florida during the 2008 Obama presidential campaign.*

# CHAPTER 2

# GET OUT OF BED AND
# FALL INTO A ROUTINE

Worn out, beat down, depressed, unhealthy, slightly overweight, horrible complexion, gray hairs at 28, binge drinker, occasional stress-smoker, single (upon the ending of my campaign romance), and unemployed. This was my new profile. Instead of relishing my accomplishing one of the most rewarding and monumental experiences of my young career in helping to get the first black man elected president of the United States and winning an enormous battleground state in Florida, I felt like crap. All around me were the faces of happy people, boasting smiles for days. I didn't know what was wrong with me. Why didn't I feel as good as everyone else around me? Why did I still feel stress instead of relief? The truth was, my mind had already moved on to worrying about what came next: the transition, and how to get myself to Washington, DC.

You see, for as far back as I can remember, I wanted to work and live in Washington, DC. I wanted to play a part in our American history, bringing change that would help people rise up, not feel pushed down. I worked as a college intern in the Florida legislature and secured an amazing gig as a legislative aide shortly after graduation. I spent the next four years of my career working for the Minority Leader of the Senate, where I learned the art of *politicking* from a sharp, petite, classy Jewish woman whom I adored.

I eventually worked my way to Congress and then landed the amazing opportunity to work on Senator Obama's campaign. It was only then that I allowed myself to dream of the day I could possibly work for the next president of the United States.

Foregoing a vacation, and in need of a steady paycheck, a week later I went back to working for Ron Klein, the Florida Congressman for whom I had been working before the start of the campaign. I was extremely grateful that he kept my job for me while I was on the campaign trail for seven months, but I didn't feel satisfied doing the same job I was doing before. I wanted more, so I worked harder. After months of hustle, countless interviews, and meetings with White House personnel, which involved flying back and forth between Florida and DC, I decided the only way I was going to get what I wanted was to move to Washington. I needed to be there, in the faces of the people I wanted something from: my dream job.

The following Monday, two days after my twenty-ninth birthday, I walked into the Florida congressional office and gave my resignation. No, I didn't have a job yet, and no, I didn't know what would happen and how I would eat for more than a few months based on the amount I had in savings, but I did it. I took a chance on myself, made the investment in myself, and moved to DC, my stress in tow.

A few months later, after working several odd jobs, I was sitting in my kitchen drinking a cup of coffee wondering what I was going to do to pay my rent the following month, stressed beyond belief, and feeling disappointed. That was when I got a call from the White House and landed my dream job. Finally, the stars had aligned, and I was going to receive a presidential appointment to work for the United States Army at the Pentagon. I couldn't believe it. I was overwhelmed with an enormous sense of honor. I was going to work amongst the best and brightest civilian and military minds in the entire world. Was I even worthy of such an opportunity? I would soon find out.

Books primed me for the difference between military and civilian culture, the length of time it took actions to go up the long chain of command, and how to navigate the surprisingly confusing building. In many ways, working in the Pentagon was similar to working on a presidential campaign. Early mornings, late evenings, and an unpredictable workday in between once again became my norm. Toward the beginning, I would find myself so consumed with work that I would miss lunch, or eat whatever I had stashed away in my desk. I started to feel as if the vicious cycle I thought I had left behind were starting all over again. That was until I was asked by a colleague if I wanted to go and check out the Pentagon Athletic Center (PAC) downstairs in the basement of the building.

For those of you wondering what it's like to work in the "Puzzle Palace" that is the Pentagon, I have two words for you: kick ass! Let's just get this out of the way—yes, it's true that there are underground roads and buildings, hidden staircases, and tons of secrets housed in the walls of the Pentagon. But what the building also has, deep underground, is a state-of-the-art facility designed for high performance, increased strength, and readiness. Anyone who works in the building could work out there for a nominal fee. Busy at all hours of the morning and well into the evening with staff and officers coming in and out, the PAC also lends itself to being a great place to network and do business.

I'll admit, what the Pentagon prep books didn't prepare me for was the culture of fitness. Working out, even during the middle of the work day, wasn't just allowed, it was encouraged. These workouts weren't mild-mannered jogs, either. Generals, admirals, and even the defense secretary worked out down there, fostering an open, brutally competitive environment.

The ratio of men to women present at the PAC was also something I noticed immediately. After agreeing to join a female colleague and friend of mine for a CrossFit workout one morning, I quickly realized that we were the only women in the entire place, and I felt like everyone was looking at us. My colleague picked up on my apprehension and the change in tone of my voice and said, "Girl, don't worry about them. Yeah, they're always going to look, that'll never change, but the fact that we're down here kicking ass, believe me when I tell you that they respect that."

I completed the hellish workout but kept thinking about her words "they respect that." It made sense: a person who respects herself by working out and taking care of herself is someone who deserves respect. But my problem for the past few years was keeping my word with myself. "I'll work out after I get home from work. I'll skip happy hour tonight and head home to cook my favorite meal." I had broken so many promises to myself at that point that I had lost count. For some reason on that day, after that particular experience, hearing those words, I decided that a major life overhaul was in order.

I had reached the point where I was ready to make the change. This is important to point out because although I had known that I needed help after almost wrecking my car from starvation and dehydration during the campaign, it wasn't until that moment in 2010 that I declared to myself that I was ready to commit to a total life reset. It was there that I decided to change all of my bad habits and make a conscious effort to reverse the years of damage and neglect on my mind and body. Of course it was going to be a bear of an undertaking, but I knew it was necessary. The first thing I started with was physical fitness. Harvard social psychologist and author Amy Cuddy (*Presence*) says, "Personal power brings us closer to our best selves, while the lack of it distorts and obscures ourselves. Power reveals."[1]

I craved something that would motivate and drive me to step completely out of my comfort zone, but give me the personal power I so desired. The only thing that made me feel like that, I soon discovered, was lifting weights in CrossFit. So, before I knew it, I had joined a CrossFit gym near my apartment with a colleague so we could hold each other accountable, and after a few weeks of making a plan and sticking to it, I found myself engaged in a sustainable and healthy routine. The motivation, encouragement, and inspiration by the people running the Pentagon changed my way of thinking for the rest of my life. I would work out at 6 a.m. four to five days a week, come home and shower, eat a healthy breakfast, grab my already prepared lunch that I had made the night before, and dash out the door heading to the office.

All it took was that first workout, and saying yes to that colleague who asked me to join him for something new and challenging. After a few months of maintaining this routine of working out in the morning, which set the tone for my day, I found myself easily rejecting anything that wasn't good for me. I cut out anything processed, fried, and filled with sugar. I replaced that extra hour of sleep each morning with a workout, and that, in turn, changed how I ate, worked, slept, and so on. I developed a way of thinking that if I was going to bust my hump at the gym in the morning, I would be damned if I was going to cancel it all out by shoving a doughnut in my mouth at our daily briefings. I said "no" to grabbing a drink after work in order to go home and cook a healthy dinner and lunch for the following day so I could get to bed in time for that early 5 a.m. wake-up call.

I maintained this routine throughout my entire assignment at the Pentagon. I won't lie to you and say that it was easy, especially when traveling all over the world and waking up in different time zones, but I did it. And when asked to resign from my post and go back to Florida to work on President Obama's reelection campaign, I vowed that if I couldn't make the same commitment to myself that I had made two years prior, I would simply turn down the opportunity.

After a lot of thought and prayer, I decided the opportunity was too important, and I accepted the offer. I made a promise to myself that if I stuck to my routine and habits, and gave it my all, leaving nothing on the table, I would make it work. I refused the thought of feeling powerless, clinging to thoughts of a potentially failed outcome, and instead focused on the process for success.

Don't let fear control your life. For most people, including myself, we show up at the doorstep of an opportunity bubbling over with anxiety and trepidation, worried about a future that hasn't yet unfolded. When you walk into a high-pressured situation in that frame of mind, you've essentially already set yourself up for failure.

Charles Duhigg, author of *The Power of Habit: Why We Do What We Do in Life and Business*, writes that after studying a young woman (Lisa) with characteristics similar to mine, scientists found that, even though her old behaviors could be tracked, her new habits had had a profound impact on her brain. This began by changing just one habit, before she began reprogramming her overall routine. In other words, changing one habit initially seemed to have a ripple effect on Lisa's other habits and, in turn, her neurological patterns.[2]

When you woke up this morning, what did you do first? Did you hop in the shower, check your email, or grab a doughnut from the kitchen counter? Did you brush your teeth before or after you toweled off? Tie the left or right shoe first? What did you say to your kids on your way out the door? Which route did you drive to work? When you got to your desk, did you deal with email, chat with a colleague, or jump into writing a memo? Salad or hamburger for lunch? When you got home, did you put on your sneakers and go for a run, or pour yourself a drink and eat dinner in front of the TV? "All our life, so far as it has definite form, is but a mass of habits," William James wrote in 1892 in *The Stream of Consciousness*.[3] Duhigg adds, "Though each habit means relatively little on its own, over time, the meals we order, what we say to our kids each night, whether we save or spend, how often we exercise, and the way we organize our thoughts and work routines have enormous impacts on our health, productivity, financial security, and happiness."[4]

Duhigg argues that each of these decisions—which are essentially habits—impacts the greater, more important aspects of our life. This way of thinking was put to the test early on during the 2012 campaign when my routine and habits came under fire. Knowing my pressure point, one of my superiors, who was also known as the office bully, messed with my workout time by throwing an assignment at me with a sixty-minute due date, literally following behind me as I left the office, threatening to fire me if I didn't participate. For me, growing up, I encountered bullies everywhere. Whether they pulled my hair on the playground, made fun of my weight and thin frame by throwing grapes at me as I ate lunch in middle school, or made up a nickname to which I didn't approve; this wasn't the first time I had come upon a bully. But I'm an adult now, so I thought all of that should have been behind me.

This wasn't the first time, or the last, where he made keeping to my routine a difficulty, but after a while I said, "enough," finding creative ways around him. I no longer feared "the bully's" threats and ignored his outbursts. His unprofessional and juvenile behavior was a reminder of what I used to tolerate from colleagues in the past. No more! You can keep putting everything and everyone else before you, or you can choose yourself. Start making exercise and healthy eating your #1 priority *right now* and don't let anyone come in between your ultimate health and happiness.

Shonda Rhimes, creator of *Grey's Anatomy* and *Scandal*, talked with Oprah about how confronting her fears and saying "yes" to things that really scared her changed her life. One of the things Shonda said yes to was health. With three daughters, she made the decision that she wanted to be around for them, and realized if she continued living the way she was, that wasn't going to happen. The result was a 110-pound weight loss. In the Oprah interview, Rhimes said, "The desire to lose weight was never about cosmetics. It was actually a byproduct of the whole thing. It wasn't the goal; it wasn't part of it. One of the yeses was, I can't say yes to everything and not say yes to taking care of myself and not say yes to health." That came only after Rhimes had an epiphany. "I work so hard at everything that I do. I work my butt off at work and I work hard at being a mother, why did I think losing weight would be easy?"[5]

## It All Starts with a Nudge

Again, some words of wisdom from Amy Cuddy:

"Just as organizations can nudge the behavior of large groups of people, individuals can nudge their own behavior towards more healthful, productive habits."[6] In other words, we can "nudge" ourselves into making healthier choices, and in doing so we can impact our overall, long-term behavior.

Stacey Colino, Health and Wellness Reporter (*US News*, About.com)—Certified Spinning Instructor, and author (*Good Food-Fast!* and *Strong Is the New Skinny*)—and I collaborated on turning her ideas on developing a routine into a set of 20 key points. We focused on straightforward advice—one main idea in each bullet—that would be particularly useful for someone with a demanding job or career, or even a busy parent getting started in developing a routine.[7]

- **Start an exercise routine first thing in the morning**. Even if it means waking up half an hour early every morning, initiate your new exercise program when you first get up. You want to be able to cross one action off your to-do list before anything has a chance to get in the way of your best-laid plans. If you plan to work out in the afternoon, a million things can come up that thwart your plans, and suddenly you're out of luck because you have no time for a workout. If you can do this first thing in the morning, your probability for success will often be much higher. Research has found that people who exercise in the morning often stick with their program and are better for it long-term. "By starting your morning with physical activity, you set the day's pace," says Cedric X. Bryant, PhD, Chief Science Officer of the American Council on Exercise. "Morning exercisers tend to stick with their exercise habit. By doing the bulk of the exercise first thing in the morning, you get your exercise in before other distractions can intrude. We can all relate to that—because once the day gets going, it's hard to get off the treadmill called life."[8]

- **Do something physical for 20–30 minutes.**

  It is helpful for someone who has a demanding job, whether it is on the campaign trail, in a company, or just a challenging work/family juggling act, to start the day with some form of exercise, even if it's 20–30 minutes. It provides you with an empowered jump start on the day. It becomes almost like a "note to self," as in, "I'm taking good care of myself today. I'm going to be strong today." That can carry on into other domains of your life, and it is powerful. When you exercise first thing in the morning, it helps you make better choices in terms of your other health habits. For example, if you started out with a 45-minute spin class or a 30-minute weight routine and a jog, why would you want to eat three doughnuts during a meeting three hours later? You will want to fuel your body as you would any other finely tuned machine.

  If your schedule prevents you from doing a physical activity first thing in the morning, that's okay. Not to worry, and don't beat yourself up. On any given day, there are plenty of opportunities to *move* throughout your workday. Here's an easy one: how about going on a "Noon Walk"—walk a mile during lunch or anytime you can carve out 30 minutes on your calendar today?

  Any form of physical activity can help you unwind and become an important part of your approach to easing stress. Make exercise a regular part of your job!

- **Just get started.**

  For most people, getting started is the hardest part. Some of it is a simple fear of the unknown, moving out of your comfort zone and into a place where you don't really know what to expect. But once you start to do something, each step will become easier than the previous. One of the truly effective measures that Stacey mentioned she has always had for herself is a 10-Minute Rule:

  > If I wake up in the morning and I am dead tired and really don't feel like exercising, I will force myself to do something active for 10 whole minutes. That is the rule. You can stand anything for 10 minutes, even if it feels terrible, you can get through 10 minutes, and chances are, about 8 minutes in—maybe even sooner—your endorphins are going to start to kick in and you will start to feel better and stronger and you think, *Oh, I could do this for another 5, 10, or 20 minutes.* Before you know it, you've got a full workout. That principle applies to initiating lots of new habits in that if you just get started and you commit to a short-term period of time, you see that you can do it and then it spurs you to keep going.[9]

- **Give it time. Keep it fresh.**

  Every individual is different when it comes to changing habits. If you are trying to change a habit such as to quit smoking or stop drinking, it may take up to

4–6 months to get over the hump, and then it takes longer to solidify it. But in terms of *starting* a habit, we can afford to be a bit more optimistic. One of the tricks to making it stick is that you have to keep the new routine "non-routine," that is, keep it interesting. You can't let it get monotonous. Allow it to get challenging continually and be creative in making it enjoyable. With fitness, just have fun with it by doing the activity with other people whose company you enjoy, or add an element of novelty by working out in a new place. Continue to keep it fresh, and that applies to anything. It's kind of like a food rut. If you eat the same healthy lunch day after day, it gets tired so you have to expand out of your comfort zone and keep it fresh. Vary what you are doing.

- **Avoid the guilt. Take time for you.**
Time is at a premium for busy people, and the logistics of scheduling—especially if there is a lack of support with childcare or supervisors not buying in to the new routine—will compound the challenge. Parents ask themselves the important question: "What am I going to do with my kids while I go to the gym for an hour?" A major factor that compounds the challenge is fatigue; it's a genuine lack of energy to exercise. Another one is guilt. For example, a lot of working parents want to go to the gym at the end of the day but are then perhaps flooded with thoughts of guilt such as, *I should instead spend time with my kids or my spouse,* and that element of guilt can

detract from their original commitment. Don't let this happen to you.

- **Mate your workout work with your job.**
  One way to avoid coming up against a challenge at work is to explain to your boss that you really need this time and that working out allows you to be your most productive self. Be positive with the facts: Working out early in the day increases your productivity and allows you to get more done. There is a benefit to the company/organization or directly to your boss; its productivity they can take to the bank. In the face of resistance, just toss it back at the boss: "Hey, since I can't do this first thing in the morning, when is a good window for me to do it instead?" Maybe there's a way to move the lunch meeting an hour later so you can go work out during lunchtime. Brand it as a workplace wellness issue and ask your supervisor for suggestions on how to make it work.

- **Make your routine a priority.**
  Making your routine #1 is very important! You have to make it a priority. You shouldn't be rigid, so allow for some flexibility because as we all know too well, life throws you curve balls all the time in whatever you're doing, so have a contingency plan. For example, if you know you just cannot work out first thing tomorrow morning, ask yourself, "When can I do this?" Try scheduling it in your smartphone or appointment book like it's a doctor's appointment. If

you do add to your electronic calendar, sync it with your work calendar to avoid scheduling meetings or appointments around that time with yourself: "I can't go to the gym tomorrow from 6 a.m. to 7 a.m. like I usually do, so after my morning meetings are over, I am going to cut out of the office from 10 a.m. to 11 a.m. and go to the gym." Make that sacred time and look for ways to make it work given the hand that you are dealt. Making your workout a priority is crucial. Think about these two things: 1.) If you don't make yourself a priority, nobody else is going to. It is totally up to you. And 2.) If you take good care of yourself, you're going to be in a better position to take care of the people around you, whether it is at work or with your family or friends. Self-care is essential and nonnegotiable because if you are unhealthy and don't have enough energy to take care of the things you have committed to in your life, you're pretty much screwed.

- **Stop making excuses and start saying "yes."**
  We always hear the excuse given when avoiding a challenge of "not having enough time." "I just don't have anyone to help me with picking up my kids, etc." or "I hate working out alone" are some common excuses. For the most part, people don't like feeling like they let someone down. If you can find a workout buddy and someone you feel accountable to, that will help you stick to it. Stacey explains, "I recently started running with a friend of mine who was training

for a race and I wanted to kick my fitness level up a notch for my wedding and so two mornings a week we would meet at 7:30 a.m. at a park near our home and run on the trail. I am confident that neither one of us would have done that had we not made that commitment to one another. We are both super busy, but our commitment was something important to one another and by making it social it became far more appealing."[10] Try something similar by joining a group exercise class, or hold a brainstorming session while going for a brisk walk with your colleagues at the office, or play softball or volleyball one weeknight or on the weekend and show the benefits of being physical together while team building.

If your challenge is figuring out who will watch your kids, maybe you trade off with a neighbor and watch each other's kids, or trade off with your spouse so that each of you is getting the benefits of that personal time to work out. Look into joining a gym that has a great childcare program, or consider buying a jogging stroller and start out fast-walking either on your own, or with a friend/neighbor who has a child of a similar age. You have to be creative if this is a priority to you. Find ways around the obstacles.

- **Schedule smart.**
  Schedule yourself more smartly. Sometimes you will have tradeoffs to face. Maybe you've decided not to go to happy hour with your colleagues because you have a yoga class you want to hit up after work instead.

Often you will have to say "no" to things in order to say "yes" to a new habit. Force yourself to do a reality check and then write down a list of the places where you feel your attention currently resides: "I don't have time to start an exercise program because 1. I have too much to do and never enough time, 2. I have young kids, 3. I am so tired all of the time and would rather get my sleep." Now go down the list and ask yourself, "Is this true?" And "How can I get around these obstacles?"

The simple act of becoming more aware of where your attention is going will help you focus it where you want it to be—on achieving your compelling goals. Too often we get distracted or caught up in unimportant tasks that end up wrecking our day and derailing our to-do lists.

The way you feel about the tasks you hate doing arc big, red flags that encourage you to find a way to pass on those un-pleasantries to someone, or something (like a system) that can tackle them for you. But first, you've gotta figure out exactly what's making you crazy in the first place.

- **Only answer crucial email first thing in the morning.**
  While you are having your morning coffee, jump on your laptop or phone and see if you have any pressing emails. If you do, take 10–15 minutes to address **only those** first thing—anything else can wait, so push everything else aside. The beauty of email is that you don't have

to answer everything when it comes in. You can push things aside until you are ready to answer them; this is a basic tool of good time management. Find a rhythm that works for you and establish a structure.

- **Eat right to avoid falling flat.**
  Eating right, especially as you start to integrate physical fitness into your routine, is extremely important and based on the individual. Some people can't stand to exercise on a full stomach; some people can't stand to exercise on an empty stomach. Stacey says, "Even when I teach a 6 a.m. spin class for 50 minutes, I can get really shaky if I haven't had anything to eat. I always have to have at least a 1 ½ cups of coffee to get me going—that is nonnegotiable. Coffee is a mental signal to myself that says 'okay, you're on now.' I usually eat half a small banana before I go spinning, and that is usually enough to boost my blood sugar, get my digestion going, and get my heart rate going. And after a morning workout I have a real breakfast that will help carry me through the day and into lunch."[11] Eating a healthy diet has to be part of the equation. Breakfast of some kind is really important. Some people don't like a lot of food in the morning, but it's important to eat something that contains complex carbohydrates, protein, and a portion of healthy fat. This is the perfect trifecta to help energize yourself for the day, and it doesn't have to be a lot. Try eating half a bagel with some almond or peanut butter and half a banana. Perhaps two eggs and sliced

avocado or a cup of yogurt with fruit is more your jam. Eat whatever it is your body can handle while working to incorporate those three key nutrients.

- **Stay fit on the road.**
You can still maintain a routine even on the road because you can take it with you. Choose to stay in hotels that have a great fitness center and stick to your routine the best way you are able. Venture out of your hotel room and sightsee by going on a brisk walk for 25 minutes in whatever city you are in and multitask that way. And always remember: when you feel and see your schedule growing more unmanageable, something is always better than nothing. The same thing goes for food. Nowadays you can find healthy food almost anywhere in the country, and you don't have to ditch your healthy eating habits just because you are traveling.

If anyone knows how challenging it is to stick to a routine when on the road, it is Congressman Tim Ryan, representative for Ohio's 13th Congressional District and author of *A Mindful Nation* and *The Real Food Revolution*. After logging thousands of miles each year, constant fundraising, being away from his wife and kids, experiencing the ever-constant environment of overactive partisanship, and feeling the stress from his job, Ryan himself began feeling like he was beginning to get burned out. So he made a change.

Like many of his House colleagues, Ryan starts most days with a cup of coffee; unlike many of them, he then spends about 45 minutes sitting in a half-lotus position—legs crossed, palms open—thinking about . . . nothing. Instead, he focuses on breathing and meditates. This, along with yoga and maintaining a healthy diet, even while on the road, helps get him through even the toughest days.

When Congress is in session, you can often find Congressman Ryan enjoying a hot yoga class at Down Dog Yoga in Georgetown, or grocery shopping and gathering wholesome, healthy foods for his work week. "Through connecting the dots among wellness, food, and mindfulness, I believe we can improve the health of our citizens and our country," says Ryan.[12]

- **Start somewhere.**
Do more today than you were doing yesterday and build from there. You can work up to any goal you set for yourself, but you must start somewhere. If you are really out of shape and unhealthy, then doing a 30-minute workout in a gym may seem like the impossible. Start out by going on a 10- to 15-minute brisk walk. This does not have to all be done at once. The key is to get started. The guideline for good health (not necessarily for weight loss) is to do 30 minutes of physical activity most days of the week, with a minimum of 4 days a week. It does not need to be 30 consecutive minutes in a day. Do three 10-minute

workouts. Do two 15-minute workouts, but make it add up to that 30-minute goal. Regardless of how long the workout is, it has to be big enough that you can still talk, but hard enough that you can't break into song.

- **Stay hydrated and drink plenty of water.**
  People often mistake thirst for hunger. You eat because you are dehydrated, and what you really need are fluids. If you don't like the taste of plain water, drink seltzer water, club soda, broth-based soup, unsweetened iced tea, and/or use a fruit diffuser or throw some fresh fruit—such as orange slices, cucumber, or lemon/lime slices—in water. Fresh fruit contains a lot of water, especially watermelon and coconut.

- **Limit your food intake after dark.**
  Don't eat a big meal at 10 p.m. and go to bed at 11 because whatever you've just eaten will sit in your stomach. Some people eat dinner at 5 or 6 p.m. and don't go to bed for a few hours later. If you usually find yourself hungry by the time you crawl into bed, it's okay to have a bit of a snack later in the evening. Make sure to keep the snack light and go for something that is not going to keep you up all night. No spicy, fatty, or fried foods, and nothing too rich, creamy, or heavy or that contains caffeine, including dark chocolate if you are sensitive. Eat in moderation in the evenings.

You should eat breakfast like a king, lunch like a prince, and dinner like a pauper. You want to front-load the day with calories and healthy nutrition while having the rest of the day to burn the calories off.

- **Prepare your meals in advance.**
Use your smartphone to keep a running grocery list. When you think of things, keep adding to it, and when you buy something, delete it. Cook a lot of staples on Sundays and then parse them out for different dishes during the week. For example, you can make a big pot of ground turkey in tomato sauce for a pasta sauce and make enough of it so you can use some of it in tacos, chili, a rice dish, or over pasta. Now you have at least three dinners for the week. Roast a bunch of vegetables that same Sunday and then parcel them out as either side dishes for something else to make during the week or combine them in different ways by adding different grains or sauces, and make different dishes; that way you don't get sick of having the same meal over and over. Be creative along the way. Roasting a whole chicken can give you enough for at least two meals that week, and three if you're cooking for one. And pre-make meals for your lunch the next day, so after your workout in the morning, you can simply grab-and-go and head to the office.

- **Have a morning ritual.**
Having a morning ritual can be extremely helpful and lends a sense of comfort in a way that feels good

as you start the day. Stacey gives this example: "My husband and I always have breakfast together even though he gets up two hours before I do. I like starting my day with him, so I will come downstairs and brew a pot of coffee and make us both breakfast while we sit and chat and read the paper together."[13] Finding an order to your morning tasks that feels good to you is important.

If you notice that you feel better when you have a healthy breakfast in the morning, you will continue making that a priority and part of your morning routine. Similarly, when you start appreciating that you have more energy when you start exercising regularly in the morning, you're going to want to keep up with that routine.

- **Take time for YOU.**
  Allowing yourself time just for you is really important. After a busy day, give yourself a wind-down period similar to that of a cool-down after a tough workout. Take a relaxing bath and let your mind wander, meditate, write in a journal, or do some general stretches. Review the highlights of the day before you go to sleep—what went right for today, what you feel good about. Try keeping a gratitude list. These activities help your mind downshift into a happier, more peaceful state of mind and set you up for a better night's sleep. Stacey discloses, "I've had trouble turning off my mind when I have had an imminent book deadline, especially if something isn't going so

well. One of the things I've gotten into the habit of doing is literally turning myself off. I will go to bed and say, 'I am going to take a vacation from worrying about this. I can deal with this in the morning.'"[14] If you defer thinking about it and you give yourself a pass in the meantime, then you allow yourself permission to think about whatever the heck you want to right now. Make it something that is calming, happy, hopeful, and optimistic. This should feel like any other form of training. You are training your mind, and this is mental discipline.

- **Don't bring your device to bed with you.**
  A lot of people bring their digital devices into the bedroom. This is not a good idea. Turn your smartphone off, but if you absolutely need to have it on, try placing it in another room. Don't bring your laptop to bed. Create boundaries; otherwise, it will suck the life out of you. You will see the difference immediately in how you start sleeping better at night. Pay close attention to the effects of these changes because they are positively reinforcing.

- **Remain motivated, and repeat.**
  You have to realize that we are all a work in progress, and the same goes for our routines. Be willing to fine-tune them, and if something isn't making a difference for you, it may be time to try something else. If you have trouble sitting still and meditating, stop meditating and turn on some music that you

like while sitting quietly and instead let your mind wander. Read a calm book or listen to music without lyrics while taking a hot bath. There are no "one size fits all" regimens for every person. This really is a process of discovery, and you have to find what works for you. This will not happen overnight, so you have to be willing to experiment. Once you find what clicks, repeat.

# CHAPTER 3

# HIGH-SPEED FUEL

## Food Is Not the Enemy

For most of my life growing up as a young girl, I was bullied for my weight and being "too skinny." I was 5'8" by the time I was in the seventh grade, and this only added to my ridiculous appearance. Most of the harassment came from female classmates, although the boys chimed in, too: "Maybe when you get some meat on your bones and grow some boobs we'll go out with you," they yelled as I passed by in the hallway. Some of the worst moments came during those awkward adolescent years of middle school. The worst was when my own teacher made a joke in front of the entire class by asking, "Are those your legs, or the drawstrings hanging out of your shorts?" I sat there in my school basketball uniform humiliated, fighting back tears while everyone laughed, including my teacher. Those moments are hard to forget, but you bury them away somewhere deep inside, hoping they won't resurface again. After years of self-reflection, I think that what it came down to was that every time someone called me "skinny," I understood it to mean "weak" or "scrawny." The word "strong" was never a word anyone used to describe me, so why would I ever think I could be strong someday?

I never paid much attention to food while growing up, because I didn't want to bring any attention to my weight. My mother cooked most nights for my father, brother, and me, and we would have dinner together at the table four to five nights a week. God bless him, but my father had so many rules at the dinner table. There was always a vegetable, finish everything on your plate, eat what your mother made for you no matter what, no complaining, and no dessert unless we did something terrific in school deserving of dessert. I ate what I was told and never really developed my own sense of appetite until college.

Only when I began doing CrossFit in 2010 did I truly come to appreciate food and what I was putting into my body and how I could use that food for fuel to get stronger, and more physically and mentally fit. Despite some common misconceptions, food is fuel. We need to change the message that we, as humans, need to eat to live, not live to eat. Finally moving past most of the childhood stuff, and accepting and changing my own eating patterns and habits, I fell in love with food.

As soon as I started CrossFit I heard people throwing the term "paleo" around, and I had no idea what they were talking about except that it involved food. Since the strongest and most well-defined athletes in my gym were self-proclaiming themselves with the title of being "paleo," I wanted to find out more. I did some of my own research, read a lot of books, and asked my coach and people at the gym a lot of questions about the rules. Before I knew it, I was reading and cooking with *Well Fed*, by Melissa Joulwan; *Practical Paleo*, by Diane Sanfilippo; and my personal favorite, *Whole30*, by Melissa Hartwig and Dallas Hartwig.

Within the first few days of my initial Paleo challenge, I felt immediate changes in my body—the most noticeable being my energy level, how naturally tired I became, and how solid I was sleeping through the night. I mean, by 8:30 p.m. I was ready for bed, lights out. My sleep dramatically improved, and I began waking up before my 5 a.m. wake-up call, full of energy and ready for my 6 a.m. CrossFit class. That same energy stayed with me all day until after dinner, and then I wanted nothing more than my pillow.

I began feeling more clear-headed, my complexion cleared up, muscles started to appear that had been buried under fat, and most important I felt great! I started to gain this surprising confidence in myself because of my appearance, how hard I was working, and the strength I was building. Eating a Paleo diet provided me with a no-nonsense approach to how and why I needed to make the best food choices, not the easiest food choices. Reading food labels more thoroughly really opened my eyes to what I had been eating previously, when I had not been paying close enough attention to the fine print and ingredients. Now, I finally felt like I was in control of the food I was eating. I was thriving, even with my crazy schedule and demanding job.

Throughout the book you're going to hear inspirational "lessons learned" from nutritionists and real-life "strength seekers" who share their recommendations and stories of what worked for them and others. I have found that Paleo and Whole30 worked for me, they're what I currently sub-scribe to and have worked for the people I have coached and advised. However, I do not want to deter anyone from doing their own reset that works for them. I want all of us to be successful in our own personal health, wellness, and balance while promoting healthy habits to others through quiet example.

I will suggest that you not put yourself through those so-called "diets" out there because they are not about establishing new preferences and habits that you can stick with in the long-term. Be aware; look for programs that are described as "resets"—that is, a short-term plan (just like a campaign) that will show you how your mind and body are affected by food and ways to create healthier habits that continue to build off of one another, creating a pyramid of strength in epic proportions.

I promise you will never go back to eating the same way again. A true reset changes your taste buds. What you once craved will no longer seem worth the calories or the way it will make you feel afterwards. Through elimination, you will find out quickly how great you feel not consuming those things.

As chef and restaurateur José Andrés explained to me, eating is the one thing (besides breathing) that we do from the moment we are born, until the day we die. Food is what we do in an enjoyment mode. You could surmise that the love a child has for its mother has to do with the amazing connection with the person who gave you love and the person who fed you first. This, in turn—whether we like it or not—in a very deep way dictates what our DNA becomes. Whether it's an aroma, smell, or faint trace of something familiar, Andrés says that people can attach that sensation to a person, a place, or a moment in time, even if it happened in some faraway place.[15]

Andrés says there have been dozens of times where a smell has brought him back to a memory of a place that he was probably too small to remember. But that scent somehow sparked a longing to know the answer to the question "Why am I so attached to this?" Growing up in a rural, farming area as he did, Andrés considers himself lucky to have been surrounded by food and in a farming community where his mom and dad cooked every day. He realized early on the power food has of evoking a memory, bringing people together, or transporting a person to another place, and he wanted to be a part of that.

Andrés also recognized an opportunity based on an unfortunate problem that runs rampant across the U.S. Americans have become extremely unhealthy, and not because of burger joints. America is unhealthy because we eat too much, and the wrong food is entirely too affordable. Perhaps someday, we are going to treat food that undermines health the same way we now treat tobacco. It's a trend that's getting momentum with proposed taxes on sugary drinks, among other initiatives.

As a result, Andrés decided that there's a need to promote more of the good things, not the bad. Andrés's desire to cover an area he felt was underexplored led him to open Beefsteak, whose motto is "real food, real quick and really good,"[16] and it now has five locations on the East Coast. In the beginning, Andrés was more in the business of opening one restaurant at a time, helping create neighborhoods while making money in the process. But then he realized, "If I serve 1,000 people at many of my restaurants a day, I know I can do good food as quick as a fast food company, so why not put the expertise to good use and serve good food fast?" He and his team asked themselves, "Can we create the next Shake Shack or Chipotle with vegetables?" He believes that while we've seen some progress with fast food companies, they're going to have to up their game because there are already chefs and restaurants that have become big competition. If more and more *healthier* establishments are created, collectively we will make them better. Andrés wants to be an agent of change and part of the solution in making Americans healthier.

Andrés recalls that moment in June 2010 when First Lady Michelle Obama called him to the South Lawn of the White House to become involved in efforts to end childhood obesity. Along with five hundred other chefs, he pledged to the First Lady and her Let's Move! Campaign his involvement in the *Chef's Move to Schools* program, run through the U.S. Department of Agriculture. To a degree, he felt he was watching history and believes that in ten or twenty years' time, this program will be as important as the Peace Corps.

Woven into his passion for healthy eating is Andrés's philosophy that food is involved in everything we do. We can explain everything in the world through food politics, wars, and of course health issues plaguing the world. Food can also help explain human evolution. It touches everything.

Given the importance of food, it is vital that great amounts of stress—whether they come from the workplace or your personal life—not impair your ability to eat well. For example, when Andrés was training under his mentor Ferran Adrià at elBulli, a Michelin 3-star restaurant near the town of Roses in Catalonia, Spain, he recalls that the kitchen was closer to a mine in its suffocating setting. Given such conditions, kitchens have long been a fairly stressful place, and having the wrong minds in a kitchen can create a negative environment for everyone else. Andrés even found himself on the receiving side of a pan-throwing chef in one kitchen. He laughs about it now, but think back to some of the worst moments you've had in your work life: emotional outbursts can take even the steadiest person into a vortex of stress.

The point is this: no matter how weak your professional or personal life may make you feel, you owe it to yourself to get as strong as possible—physically, psychologically, and emotionally. The physical strength, of course, comes from a combination of eating well and maintaining good physical fitness (in Andrés's case, he exercises on the elliptical machine five to six days a week), while the psychological and emotional strength often comes from pursuing activities you enjoy. As Andrés shared with me, in his free time he

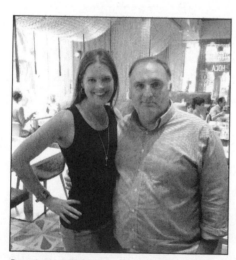

*Laurie A. Watkins and José Andrés at his restaurant Jaleo in Washington, DC.*

enjoys scuba diving, traveling, tending to his minigarden at home, and taking his annual trip to Spain, where he enjoys exploring new and old parts of his beloved country with his wife. The only time he allows himself to watch television is between seven and eight o'clock in the morning, while on the machine. Do whatever works for *you*: just start moving, and keep going. You'll stimulate endorphin production—and that's an automatic "happy rush" that will leave you feeling strong and accomplished.

## Crash and Burn

Jamie Leeds, chef and owner of Hank's Oyster Bar and the JL Restaurant Group in Washington, DC, knows all too well about stress while working around food.[17] Leeds avoided a fast approaching and potentially deadly crash and burn just before finally making the decision to change her life and ultimately lose 165 pounds. Leeds, a self-taught chef in her midtwenties, began her career in the kitchen of Union Square Café in New York City, where owner Danny Meyer (Shake Shack) promoted her from line cook to sous-chef in just under a year. Meyer then sent his protégée to Europe to train at such prestigious establishments as the Hotel Negresco in Nice, Pain Adour et Fantaisie in Grenade-sur-l'Adour, and Gascogne and Hostellerie du Cerf in Belgium.

After working for Meyer for four years, Leeds worked to create menus and organize restaurant kitchens in New York, San Francisco, and Chicago. In 1997, she became the chef of The Globe in New York, and in 2000 she joined forces with the Myriad Restaurant Group as a corporate consulting chef, where she traveled the country opening restaurants like the famed Steelhead Grill in Pittsburgh and Earth & Ocean in Seattle.

Traveling the country and working in a kitchen are physically demanding jobs. People often work in very high heat; they endure nonstop, time-sensitive situations; and they constantly lift heavy pots, crates of vegetables, and large sides of beef—all within a kitchen that is already a stressful environment.

Leeds loved food and struggled with weight her entire life; up and down constantly, it was a battle of losing and gaining, losing and gaining. Over the years she had become a stress eater, and the consequences of constantly working in stressful conditions in the kitchen brought on binge eating—not the best way to get her "fuel." It got even worse after she opened her first restaurant as executive chef and owner of the 65-seat Hank's Oyster Bar in May 2005. With lines out the door the moment it opened, she performed jobs an executive chef wouldn't normally do, like working the fry station and shucking oysters whenever necessary. The restaurant was very successful, but for Leeds, more success brought more stress to her body. She ate standing up, putting in her mouth whatever was handy when she had a moment. On days off, she felt totally exhausted and didn't want to cook anything, not even for herself. This led to grabbing anything that was close by, usually something quick and unhealthy.

Over the course of the next few years, the physical demands of the kitchen really took its toll on Leeds. She began to gain more weight, and as the years went on, her knees got to the point where it was so painful she could barely walk. Leeds recalls having to take one step at a time going up the stairs and needing to hang onto the wall for support because the pain was so excruciating. At first it was her knees, which got so depraved that she developed osteoarthritis, resulting in meniscus tears in both knees that required surgery. This went on for a couple of years, and her quality of life went to hell. All she wanted to do was be horizontal, all the time. She couldn't even run and play with her son any longer. On the social side of things, you can imagine how lonely and isolated she became. Pain had begun running Leeds's life.

After trying again and again to lose the weight, she finally got to the point where she said to herself, "I don't want my life to be this way. This is not me. This is not who I am." Something had to change. Leeds's orthopedic surgeon suggested she have double knee replacement surgery. After leaving the doctor's office, she began to think about what a double knee surgery would look like from the perspective of a chef whose success depended on her being able to move freely throughout a kitchen, and then she began to consider alternatives.

The root cause of Jamie's pain was from being overweight, which eventually stripped her body of the muscle it needed to support her frame. A friend of Leeds mentioned a weight loss surgery called DS (duodenal switch). Deciding she had nothing to lose, Leeds attended informational seminars and did extensive research on the long-term effects of such an invasive and irreversible procedure. DS is the most extreme of the bariatric surgeries because the band cannot be removed or stretched.

Leeds went for it. It was a life-altering measure that helped her to do a 180-degree flip in terms of health and fitness. She was almost three hundred pounds, and 5'9". She lost 165 pounds within an eighteen to twenty-four-month period. The most surprising change for Jamie was that all that pain she had felt day in and day out had all but disappeared. Before the surgery, Leeds was prediabetic, and had high blood pressure and cholesterol levels. Suddenly after the surgery, all her levels went down and returned to normal. Leeds became happier. She regained the physical ability to move and became motivated to get out of the house and socialize in order to meet people and expand her business. Needless to say, she never ended up needing to have both of her knees replaced. Changing her diet and portion size and regaining the ability to exercise and do the activities she once loved reopened her eyes to the reality of living a healthy and well-balanced life.

Since the surgery, Jamie has opened four additional restaurants and a bar and is currently working on a project along The Wharf in the heart of Washington, DC. Jamie is on a trajectory to build her company and take it to places she never dreamed of but admits that had she not lost the weight, changed her diet and entire outlook on eating, and become a happier and healthier person, none of what she has created would have happened. Jamie admits to having low self-esteem her entire life from consistently being overweight and says that even after losing the weight, you just don't immediately snap out of that. Having a solid support system around you is a critical component for success, so don't be afraid to ask for help.

Jamie's life improved not only professionally, but socially, as well. Every few weeks, Jamie would have to buy new pants, letting go of the past and eventually her entire wardrobe because it no longer fit. She took it slow, fully embracing the new energy she felt, and soon began to take on more with her fitness and lines of business. She began going out on dates, a lot more dates than she had ever gone on before. Jamie's entire life changed, and for the first time ever, women were asking her for her phone number instead of the other way around. Her confidence skyrocketed, and that self-assurance helped her with everything else—meeting and marrying the love of her life, Tina, developing a closer relationship with her son, Aiden, expanding her businesses, and most important creating and living the life she always wanted.

Short-term diets don't address your habits, or relationship with food, only your current intake. I'm here to tell you that changing your eating habits permanently is the only way to make long-lasting changes to your metabolism. These types of permanent changes don't just happen overnight or even with one decision to make a change to your life. It takes weekly and daily choices to make lifestyle changes.

In other words, the improvements in Jamie's life would not have happened had she not continued to eat properly after her surgery. Now, Leeds stays healthy by eating a very nutrient- and protein-focused diet. All of her meals contain one protein and vegetable(s), and she focuses on using spices for enhanced flavor. She has lightened up the dishes in her restaurants, as well—no more butter and cream sauces, but instead relishes and salsas. Leeds is a big fan of dry rubbing and marinating meats to increase the flavor of the dish instead of adding unnecessary fat. She also eats a lot of oysters, which are surprisingly healthy—packed with protein and tons of zinc. Plus, a dozen oysters are only 110 calories!

According to Jamie, eating well also involves making a plan for how to attack each day. Therefore, it's important to know your schedule for the day. Leeds always eats a good breakfast in the morning, which usually consists of granola, yogurt, a protein shake, and an occasional bagel on the weekends if she uses that as her "cheat" for the week. For lunch, Jamie will have grilled shrimp, or a piece of fish and a salad. Leeds's family is her number-one priority, and she works hard at trying to get home at a reasonable hour to cook and eat dinner together. A typical dinner for the Leedses could be a piece of grilled fish, seafood, or a mixture of grilled shrimp with beets, avocado, cucumber, tomatoes, and basil. There is always a side of fresh greens, since the family loves big, crunchy salads with a lot of stuff in them. But Leeds admits that when she needs a go-to meal, she always goes for sashimi, simple raw fish, often sliced very thin, which is her favorite, and very healthy.

Yet just like Andrés acknowledged, Leeds recognizes that her strength doesn't only come from eating right. She has also gained emotional strength by believing in herself. Though Leeds has over two hundred employees for whom she's responsible, she maintains an amazing sense of self-assurance that everything will work out. "I just know that everything will be okay. I have faith in myself and tremendous support from the people around me who lift me up." Leeds recommends creating a support system around you. Whether you choose to go to therapy, consult a trainer, or hire a babysitter, you can't do it alone. It's impossible to be successful on your own. You have to recruit people around you, and if you don't have the money, then ask friends. Don't be afraid to reach out to someone and ask for help. You can't do this kind of thing alone. None of us can.

*To enjoy Jamie Leeds's famous Oyster Stew Recipe (for 4), see page 190.*

## Slow and Steady Wins the Race

Are you familiar with the expression "There's no such thing as a free lunch"? Although most people are familiar with the phrase, I bet you've never seen the kind of carnage I'm talking about—campaign staffers waiting in line, legs twitching, ready to tear into the kitchen, ripping apart as many pieces of pizza out of the box as their hands would carry. I've witnessed folks go nuts, consuming as much as they could get their hands on, simply because it was free. And what's crazy is that not too long ago, I used to be just as guilty as the next guy. Half the time I wasn't even hungry or had dinner plans immediately following an event, yet you would find me off in the corner shoving five or six crab cakes and egg rolls in my mouth.

Did I really believe my skills were so incredibly stealthy that no one ever saw me shoving a shrimp or dumpling into my mouth as I turned around pretending to talk to the invisible person behind me?! Oh, please! I had done it so many times, I was sure my secret was safe. The problem was, I started believing my own lies and immediately upon leaving an event would forget how many mini sliders I had consumed, making it difficult later when trying to calculate how many minisliders make up one traditional cheeseburger. Tired of the same greasy food, I learned to change my life and removed those extra pounds by learning to say "no, thank you" at events and receptions and holding onto a glass of club soda instead.

Apparently, I'm not alone. According to Lori Garver, former NASA Deputy Administrator, she is well-known for the "club soda reception," which she learned from her mom.[18]

Garver said she always had aides around her who knew to switch out the glass of white wine she had been nursing with club soda. You have to have a strategy on how to manage yourself at these kinds of events, because the frequency with which they come is mind-boggling.

I'll share a little secret with you: of all the industries I was in, the aerospace industry hosts the best events, with the best food. I especially loved hanging with the space geeks, because they liked to dance all night. All events and meetings involved food, and a majority if not all of the events involved alcohol. Pigs in a blanket, cheese cut into little cubes, meat carving stations, fondue towers would stare you right in the face saying, "Eat me, I'm free!" Just ask my friend Phil Larson, who worked at the White House and admitted to attending at least 1,000 receptions over the course of one year, and sometimes as many as six or seven on any given workday.[19]

It took Phil, former White House senior advisor and then communications mastermind for Elon Musk at Space X, and now assistant dean at the University of Colorado Boulder, many receptions to figure out he had to change his form of fuel. In May 2014 while we were both at a space symposium in Colorado Springs, we decided to head over to the nearby Garden of the Gods during some downtime for a moderate hike in the mountains. Out of shape, winded, and looking to me for relief, he gasped, "Stop, I can't breathe, and my lungs are on fire." Right then and there, he proclaimed to me and to himself, "I can't do this anymore. I have to make a change." With my help and a nutrition plan consisting of a strict Paleo diet, moderate exercise, and increased

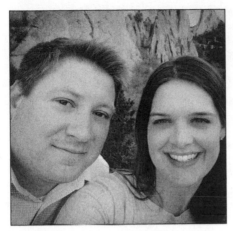

*Phil Larson and Laurie A. Watkins, Garden of the Gods, Colorado Springs, CO.*

sleep, Larson lost thirty-five pounds and learned how to create a better work-life balance for himself while working in the White House.

## The Day of Phil's Awakening

But before there was sun-shine, there was rain. Phil was a mess. Attending on average six to seven events every day, which could range anywhere from a breakfast to a luncheon to a roundtable and then three or four happy hours that he would hop between, was the norm for him. And most nights, he would go back to the office after the events ended just to play catch-up on work. It was business as usual at the White House to grab lunch and eat at your desk (if you were lucky), but most days lunch was consumed in a meeting or even walking in the hallway on the way to another meeting.

After a few years of living a fast and high-functioning lifestyle, Phil cracked. He told himself no more putting it off and trying to get to the next milestone job or career advancement before doing something to change his diet. In the past, the only time Phil ever took time for himself had been in between jobs. Cashing in his leftover vacation time before going on to the next job had been his MO. But Phil quickly realized that even with a ninety-day "sabbatical" here and there, it was never going to make up for all the missed home-cooked, healthy meals, and hours of sleep.

Phil asked me for help that day on the rock at Garden of the Gods, and I took it seriously because I could see that he was unhappy, suffering, and struggling to keep it all together. I feel fortunate that I was the person he came to looking for results because in just thirty short days he was able to show real gains in progress and weight loss—no more aches and pains, no more getting winded going up and down the stairs at work, and he felt great.

The Paleo reset worked well for Phil because he saw quick results, and most important, he saw everything else in his life improve: sleep, increased energy, lower stress level, and weight loss. He recalls coworkers laughing because some thought it was just a fad diet. Some colleagues were more supportive than others, but they all noticed changes in him within just a month. Colleagues remarked that he was more cogent in meetings, offering good ideas in a clear and concise manner. Phil Larson was a new man: he suddenly felt like he had a clearer sense of purpose, and he felt more jovial and charismatic among colleagues and friends. After consistently feeling better when he woke up each day, he realized that he'd been caught in a deadly spiral. Work had been causing him to be unhealthy, which in turn caused him not to be optimal at work.

People in the office began to refer to him as "Paleo Phil," so at times it became kind of fun. The surprising part was that changing his diet to Paleo actually turned out to be sustainable, which was key for him. Admittedly, Phil is not the kind of person who prepares his lunch at home and brings it to work. He tried it a few times and it just didn't work for him, so instead Phil would make smart choices at the White House cafeteria, where he ate lunch most days during the work week.

Phil learned quickly that while taking on a reset was a challenging process, it also brought changes in social interactions, too. When out at restaurants, Phil says he felt like he had become "that guy" who said "yes, I'll have a burger with no bun, no cheese, nothing, plain" and not batting an eyelash when people tried to tear him down. He wasn't just ordering club soda during happy hours anymore, but he was also fielding questions about why he wasn't drinking, dealing with peer pressure to just have "one."

During the first thirty days of his new diet, Phil observed that people like to talk about two things with colleagues: the weather and dieting. If people think you're on a diet, they are going to bring it up and talk about it, and just like with anything in politics, you have to give the straight answer and move on and not let it bother you. And in Phil's case, once that happened and people started seeing results, they were astounded and made comments like, "Wow, it's actually working."

Social support is going to be mission critical to your reset, especially from those you spend the most time with—colleagues, family, and friends. Don't feel nervous about telling people that you're doing a reset, and let them know how they can be supportive. It could sound like this:

Talking to Your Partner/Spouse: "My cravings are out of control, and I'm not happy with myself. This is going to be a challenge, but I need you to support me by not offering me wine, sweets, or things not included in my reset. I really want to see this through. Can you agree to that and remain supportive?"

Talking to Your Coworkers: "I'm dragging these days and want to feel more alert, and be more productive. I think this new nutrition program is going to make me sleep better, reset faster, and give me more energy. It'll be tough to pass on the office birthday party cake and ice cream, but I have to commit to this 100%, or I won't know if it's working. Cool?"

Phil's new diet led to better sleep patterns and the ability to wake up in the morning with more energy. He started to feel like everything around him was improving, not just his waistline. His experience was that within the first week or two of a strict Paleo diet, he had an enormous sense of energy, even without the coffee on which he'd become dependent. His new diet left his body running more efficiently, with fewer aches and pains. Feeling less pain led to the increase in his desire and ability to exercise more regularly.

To address the oral fixation with things like chips, popcorn, or gum, none of which are Paleo, Phil learned to try almonds, cashews, or walnuts as convenient snacks at the office. He advises that you drink water throughout the day, and if you need to switch things up, try club soda or add lemons and limes to your water bottle, but absolutely no soda. Phil recommends treating yourself to fresh items from the market; you might think you're spending more for food, but as you shrink your waistline, keep in mind that you're eating less and less often.

Dearly missing the carbs and pasta that were a huge favorite for Larson and something he used to eat often for dinner before going Paleo, he learned to make spaghetti and meatballs, substituting spaghetti squash for pasta, creating his own **arrabiata sauce and meatball recipe** (see pages 191-192) that includes cauliflower rice instead of breadcrumbs. Phil recommends that you always make enough meatballs to keep some stashed away in the freezer for those times when you need an emergency protein to add to a stew, soup, eggs, greens, or some steamed vegetables. And if you're a social person who likes to have people over, the meatballs are an excellent recipe that will keep you honest even while you play host to happy guests who will ask for your recipe.

## Don't Eat the Cake

During the 2012 presidential campaign, a friend and colleague from back home in DC thought I was feeling a bit homesick, so he sent me a little something to brighten my day. After a long meeting, listening to some of my colleagues argue back and forth over a major strategy decision, I headed back toward my cube, looking forward to putting my headphones in and drowning out the sound of their bickering with some music. When I rounded the corner, I noticed a crowd congregating around my desk.

"What's so interesting over there?" I asked. A small crowd of staffers parted like the sea, allowing me to see what it was they were all staring at.

Sitting next to my laptop on my desk was a large, bright, pink box with the words "Georgetown Cupcake" splashed across the front. The staffers swirled around it silently like sharks. They were all looking at me with big round eyes, mouths salivating at the hopes of getting one of those delicious cupcakes in their hands. I couldn't help but laugh out loud. Obviously I wasn't going to eat a dozen cupcakes. I was in the middle of a thirty-day *Paleo challenge* with my new gym and didn't dare cheat, so I quickly decided to share every cupcake in the box with my colleagues. I forced them to cut them in half, maximizing the share for everyone surrounding the box. After that, I was a major hit with the staff and never got a complaint when asked to pitch in on an assignment. My strategy there was to avoid throwing them away, sharing what I couldn't eat, but not *passing the fat* entirely onto someone else. I divided the treats among the team, and everyone was happy.

Christy Adkins, one of the most respected and decorated women in the sport of CrossFit, admits that the nursing profession she works in has a bad tendency to celebrate every birthday (which is almost every day) with a cake, cookie, pie, or cupcake.[20] These frequent celebrations grew challenging where she worked, and to avoid being seen as rude every time she refused, Adkins let everyone at work know that while she was happy to celebrate their "day," she couldn't eat the sweets but would make an exception when it was her time for celebration. This simple task relieved a lot of pressure for Adkins with her colleagues and opened up dialogue about the benefits of not eating the cake every single time.

Whether at home or in the office, social support, especially in person and from those with whom you spend the most time, is important when making a major change and breaking old patterns. It's up to you to start the conversation. Maybe that means asking your boss or supervisor if you can adjust your work start or end time to accommodate the hours of operation at your gym or asking management for a water dispenser in the break room for all employees to use. Maybe it means having a conversation with the person in the office in charge of doing the catering order for morning meetings requesting no more trays piled high with doughnuts, muffins, and pastries because eating that stuff every day isn't good for *anyone*.

The one thing I try to remember in order to be a good communicator is that people are not mind readers. You have to ask people for help and support. You can't expect people to know what you need, when you need encouragement or even a pat on the back. But if you explain to folks what you're doing, why it's so important, and how they can help, you dramatically increase the probability of your own success.

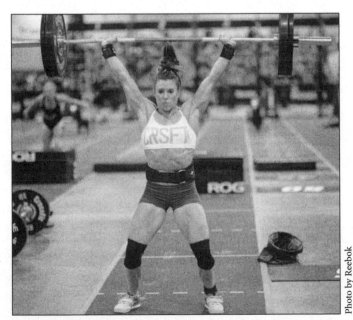

*Christy Adkins competing at the 2016 Reebok CrossFit Games Atlantic Region*

Photo by Reebok

Adkins didn't always eat, sleep, or take care of herself the way she does now.[21] She admits she was still very much living in "party mode" after graduating from college in 2008. She had her job, she had her own training, and she was a personal trainer at a gym advocating a healthy lifestyle to her clients, yet she still wasn't completely taking care of herself. That was until her friend Melody introduced her to The Zone, and she started paying attention to the macronutrients and whether each meal she ate contained a protein, a carbohydrate, and a healthy fat. Within weeks Adkins's body composition changed, and her training brought other exciting milestones simply from changing her diet. She began to see her abdominal muscles defined. She also did her first strict pull-up six months after starting and admits that even when she played varsity lacrosse at George Washington University, she was never able to do a strict pull-up and feels the new diet had a lot to do with that.

Now that she is a full-time, competitive athlete who travels a great deal, she offers advice to other professionals with hectic lifestyles that keep them on the road. Christy recommends holding yourself accountable by deciding ahead of each trip—whether it be for work or fun—which foods you are not going to allow yourself to eat. For example, if you know you will be gone for five days on a work trip, try and make a commitment to yourself that for four of those five days you will not consume alcohol or dessert at dinner. Then, while looking at your work calendar ahead of time, decide "Okay, for this particular work dinner, I am going to allow myself a cocktail or glass of wine and/or dessert at dinner." For the rest of that week, though, stay committed to the promise you made with yourself ahead of time, remaining true to your diet or regimen.

## Backyard Garden

Throughout his childhood, Bill Nye grew up always having something green (beans, peas) with dinner, along with a salad.[22] He sees some of his colleagues at dinners or luncheons ingest food in a way that is "just wild," as if it were their last meal. Always eating pretty well, Bill was motivated to build his own backyard garden in Los Angeles, California. Along with the kale and fennel that he grows, his garden also has a bunch of asparagus, strawberries, tomatoes, fresh herbs, and the most delicious oranges and grapefruits.

Sometimes there is such an overabundance of fruits and veggies that Bill invites the neighbors over to pick what they like. Most of the time he has more oranges and grapefruits than he can eat or knows what to do with. And when he's in L.A., he makes sure to have both an orange and a grapefruit every single morning for breakfast, fresh off the trees out back.

Growing fruits and vegetables seems overwhelming to most people, but it's actually much simpler than it sounds (plus, you don't have to trade in your suburban or urban lifestyle for a life in the sticks in the name of self-sufficiency or savings). All you need is a few square feet of the great outdoors, a water source, and a little time. Your grandparents did it, and so can you, according to health educators Liza Barnes and Nicole Nichols, who coauthored "The Benefits of Growing Your Own Food" for Sparkpeople.com.[23]

If you still aren't convinced, consider these benefits of backyard gardening:

- **Improve your family's health.**
  Eating more fresh fruits and vegetables is one of the most important things you and your family can do to stay healthy. When they're growing in your backyard, you won't be able to resist them, and their vitamin content will be at their highest levels as you bite into them straight from the garden. Parents, take note: A study published in the *Journal of the American Dietetic Association* in 2013 found that preschool children who were almost always served homegrown produce were more than twice as likely to eat five servings of fruits and vegetables a day— and to like them more—than kids who rarely or never ate homegrown produce.[24]

- **Save money on groceries.**
  Your grocery bill will shrink as you begin to stock your pantry with fresh produce from your backyard. A packet of seeds can cost less than a dollar, and if you buy heirloom, nonhybrid species, you can save the seeds from the best producers, dry them, and use them next year. If you learn to dry, can, or otherwise preserve your summer or fall harvest, you'll be able to feed yourself even when the growing season is over.

- **Reduce your environmental impact.**
  Backyard gardening helps the planet in many ways. If you grow your food organically, without pesticides and herbicides, you'll spare the earth the burden of

unnecessary air and water pollution, for example. You'll also reduce the use of fossil fuels and the resulting pollution that comes from the transport of fresh produce from all over the world (in planes and refrigerated trucks) to your supermarket.

- **Get outdoor exercise.**
  Planting, weeding, watering, and harvesting add purposeful physical activity to your day. If you have kids, they can join in, too. Be sure to lift heavy objects properly, and to stretch your tight muscles before and after strenuous activity. Gardening is also a way to relax, destress, center your mind, and get fresh air and sunshine.

- **Enjoy better-tasting food.**
  Fresh food is the best food! How long has the food on your supermarket shelf been there? How far did it travel from the farm to your table? Comparing the flavor of a homegrown tomato with the taste of a store-bought one is like comparing apples to wallpaper paste. If it tastes better, you'll be more likely to eat the healthy, fresh produce that you know your body needs.

- **Build a sense of pride.**
  Watching a seed blossom under your care to become food on your and your family's plates is gratifying. Growing your own food is one of the most purposeful and important things a human can do—it's work that

directly helps you thrive, nourish your family, and maintain your health. Caring for your plants and waiting as they blossom and "fruit" before your eyes provides an amazing sense of accomplishment!

- **Stop worrying about food safety.**
  With recalls on spinach, tomatoes, peanut butter, and more, many people are concerned about food safety in our global food marketplace. When you responsibly grow your own food, you don't have to worry about contamination that may occur at the farm, manufacturing plant, or transportation process. This means that when the whole world is avoiding tomatoes, for example, you don't have to go without—you can trust that your food is safe and healthy to eat.

- **Reduce food waste.**
  Americans throw away about $600 worth of food per person, each year! It's a lot easier to toss a moldy orange that you paid $0.50 for than to dump a perfect red pepper that you patiently watched ripen over the course of several weeks. When it's "yours," you will be less likely to take it for granted and more likely to eat it (or preserve it) before it goes to waste.

## Think of Your Body as a Bank Account

Think of your body as a bank account and forget about counting calories. Your ticket to a lean, healthy body is eating

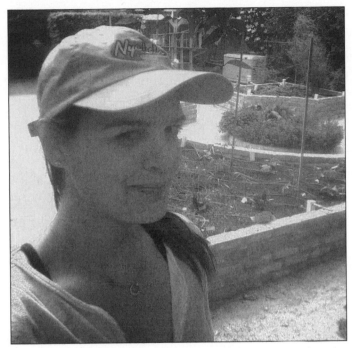

*Laurie A. Watkins tending to the fruits and vegetables in Bill Nye's home garden, Los Angeles, CA.*

*clean.* That means embracing foods like vegetables, fruits, and healthy proteins and fats. It also means cutting back (or in my recommendation, eliminating) dairy, refined grains, added sugars, salt, and unhealthy fats. In my analogy, it goes like this: Clean food = money, and the more *clean* food you deposit into your bank account, the more money you have to spend. So if *dirty* food = a withdrawal from your bank account, then that means every time you eat dirty food, you have less money to play with or spend, and less clean food in your account to cover any emergencies or rainy-day activities like "cheat meals."

For anyone who hasn't made a deposit of clean food in a very long time, well, you can imagine how long that person has carried a negative balance with him- or herself. My hope is to catch you before you hit bankruptcy. It is possible, and just like with any bankruptcy "relief assistance program," you will have to work hard at eliminating the debt, following the rules of the program or risk default. Eventually, you will be able to create some cash reserve, climbing out of the hole you have felt buried in, no longer allowing food to control you, and witnessing real results.

If we're going to be realistic, we have to take into consideration any sudden stressors that will probably come up, as they tend to do. This is life. But it's important to know what your coping plan will look like when there is a death in the family, a break-up, bad news at work, or just a straight-up bad day.

Will you go back to your reset, perhaps because it feels comfortable and gives you control during a time when you feel your life is out of control? Will you hold off going full-throttle, leaving room for certain slips and triggers, remaining true to the program's foundational principles, and eventually planning on a full reset? Or will you give up completely, turning your life back over to your grief and stress, continuing to live the life you don't want? Only you can make the decision, and that will depend on how bad you want it, and how committed you are to the process.

If you eat foods like lean protein, good-for-you carbohydrates and fats, fresh fruits, and vegetables five to six times a day in the right amounts; drink lots of water; and exercise regularly, I guarantee you will turn your sluggish metabolism into a fat-burning machine. That bank account I talked about earlier will be full and overflowing in abundance if you follow this advice:

1. Eliminate Processed Foods
2. Bump up your Veggies
3. Cut Down on Saturated Fats
4. Eliminate/Reduce Alcohol Intake
5. Un-Sweeten Your Diet
6. Hold the Salt
7. Reduce/Eliminate Dairy
8. Eat Good-for-You Proteins and Fats
9. Up Your Fruit Intake
10. Nix Refined Grains

In truth, I did not always eat like this, and it took me working at the Pentagon and being a part of a culture that supported and encouraged people to take care of themselves not just mentally, but also physically, to get to the point that I could fully stand up for myself and say, "Yes, this is a priority to me, and I will work hard and around whatever I need to in order to accomplish this task daily." Feeling supported by a culture that promoted and prescribed wellness and being at the top of your game gave me a clear snapshot of what an organization dedicated to greatness looks like. It starts at the top. When leadership and management see the importance and benefits of wellness, it flows all the way down the chain of command, affecting the entire organization.

I want to feel good and don't want to feel bad about doing so. I eat really clean the majority of the time and subscribe to an 80/20 (80%/20%) Paleo/Whole30 diet, 365 days a year.

Eighty/twenty means that I stick to my Paleo/Whole30 regimen eighty percent of the time and allow myself the opportunity to consume things not in my program only twenty percent of the time. The twenty percent *could* include things like dairy, alcohol, sugar, grains, carbohydrates, beans, and basically everything not included in the Paleo/Whole30 guidelines. Through my first reset, I discovered that soy did not agree with my body. It was only through the elimination and eventual reintegration of soy into my diet that I realized it had been a trigger to breakouts and skin irritations on my face.

My recommended program includes lean meat; fresh fish; a ton of veggies, fruit, nuts, and seeds; and tons of essential fats, whether it's avocado, coconut oil, or light olive oil. I eat medium-sized meals and snack in between. I suggest my clients follow the same, what I call the 80/20 rule. Eighty percent of the time they should follow the guidelines to a reset very closely, and 20 percent of the time they're free to loosen up and just eat what they want to eat. There's a lot more to life than worrying about food and calories. I believe that, in some cases, it's better to eat the wrong food with the right mindset and awareness.

Unfortunately, the 80/20 rule doesn't apply to those dealing with serious health challenges or allergies or intolerances to specific foods. It's never a good idea for someone with Hashimoto's disease and gluten intolerance, for example, to just throw caution to the wind and have a carbohydrate feast. That could trigger an immune reaction lasting up to several weeks. Be smart! The purpose of a reset is to identify and exclude foods that may be causing an adverse effect in a person, after which those foods are reintroduced one at a time, and slowly.

## Bite to Eat

During the 2012 presidential campaign, I had to slightly adjust my program by allowing myself to snack more often. The major difference between me and most of my colleagues was the food they were choosing to eat, or snack on, and the size of the "snack" they ate. My cup of nuts or dried fruit snack would easily be undermined by my deskmate, torturing me with his quarter-pound burger grilled to perfection, gently nestled in between a delicious potato roll, covered in cheese, and topped with bacon and a gooey sauce.

If you're Bill Nye, you snack on apples, or apples and nut butter (sunflower, almond, or cashew nut butter). Raw, unsalted nuts are also a good source of protein, vitamin E, magnesium, and zinc and are easy to grab-and-go or keep in your bag as a backup if you're traveling that day and run into a situation where you have to wait to get to good food. Avocados—filled with nutrients, vitamins, potassium, and heart-healthy fatty acids—are another favorite fruit of Bill's. Since he started incorporating these into breakfast and lunch, he has noticed positive benefits, including reduced inflammation in his joints and a better feeling regarding his overall health. Slice half an avocado as you would an apple, sprinkle it with sea salt, and you have a great snack you can eat sitting at your desk.

Back on the campaign, I never really ate out unless I had to. My walk to "grab food" with colleagues was often a coffee run. Instead of buying food, I would treat myself to an iced coffee (always black, unsweetened) or iced tea, avoiding the pressure, but still being social with my team. Most nights I would make enough dinner to have as the next day's lunch and snacks. I used a Crock-Pot to cook protein during the day, grilled fish and steak a few nights a week, and roasted whole chickens from time to time just to have the meat in a container in the fridge to easily throw on a salad or with my eggs the next morning. It was usually 9 p.m. or so before I would get home from the office, but I would still turn on the grill for dinner and cook the shrimp that had been marinating all day. It takes a lot of work, dedication, and time, but it gets easier when you create a routine. Some people don't think it's possible, but that's probably because they've never tried it. Some people don't believe in the lifestyle and think that you must be doing something that unnaturally takes you to where you are, like a *magic* diet pill or plastic surgery. Otherwise, they believe, you would have failed.

If you make the commitment to change, and prioritize your life accordingly, you will and can succeed. Every Sunday when I wasn't traveling the state, I would create my own personal menu for the week. I would look at how many nights I would be in town vs. how many nights were spent on the road, and I would plan my grocery shopping accordingly. It's really not that much more expensive to eat clean. I would plan and budget (this sucked, because I had to constantly remind myself of the significant pay cut I took to come work on the campaign) and try really hard to buy only the things I needed to eat vs. what I desired to eat and wouldn't have time to eat before my next trip, wasting food and money.

Here is a simple list of go-to healthy snacks that will satisfy you throughout the day. Whether you're traveling or simply heading out the door to the office or school, you can easily throw any of these into your work/gym bag, or bring them from your own kitchen in preparation for a business trip, all TSA compliant (besides the hummus, salsa, and dressing):

- Tangerines, apples, bananas
- Prepackaged microgreens with a side of dressing
- Apple slices and single-serving nut butter containers
- Small container of berries or dried fruit
- Protein bars that are sugar-, dairy-, gluten-, grain-, and legume-free (e.g., peanut-free)
- Carrot sticks and single-serving hummus containers
- Celery and nut butter
- Mixed nuts and seeds
- All-natural meat sticks
- Plantain chips and guacamole/salsa

Austin Willard, a cadet at West Point, has this approach to food, and in this particular order:

Food is fuel. Food is the fuel necessary to perform at a high level. We all have to consume food, so it's an opportunity to sit down, take a break, and spend time with people. Food is also there to enjoy, to savor.[25] Willard feels that a lot of people get that order confused. When it becomes primarily "Is this going to taste good?" over "Who do I get to eat it with?" or "Is this actually going to fuel me at all?" that's when you have a problem. Especially in light of grueling training missions, Willard had to adopt the mentality "This is fuel even if it tastes terrible" and "If this is the fuel necessary to do what I need to do, then I'm going to eat it." But don't go too far and lose your ability to enjoy food. It is okay to treat yourself to ice cream or chicken wings after you accomplish something major, but it's not okay to eat those things in abundance and as part of your regular diet. Reward yourself when you've earned the treat.

People need to treat themselves periodically in their diet, or they eventually face that moment when they're so hungry they binge on anything they can get their hands on, mostly foods high in fat and calories. For me, my weakness is good pizza, and a really good burger, and when I get a sugar craving, it's usually for ice cream or a doughnut. Let me be clear—I am not perfect 100 percent of the time. I pride myself on eating an 80/20 diet, that is, a program that involves eating clean, healthy foods 80 percent of the time and that gives me the freedom to indulge in anything else 20 percent of the time. When I do reward myself with a "cheat," you better believe it's going to be worth it. A cheeseburger with a bun and fries, real cheesecake, or an Italian cannoli— that's what I'm willing to cheat for, not a prepackaged TastyKake. I learned to savor my food more, and eating out has turned into more of a celebration (as José Andrés talks about in the beginning of this chapter), versus something I used to do a few times a day. I grew to truly appreciate food and its purpose to fuel the body. I accepted and eventually became proud of the fact that I learned to cook for myself when I had no one else to cook for. Now I'll cook for anyone willing to eat a healthy meal. And leftovers reign king in our household.

## Let's Go!

To get you started, Elissa Goodman, Certified Holistic Nutritionist who works with people from all walks of life to help cleanse their bodies and their lives, offers expert recommendations for everything from energy-boosting snacks to "brain food" boosters that will turn your slump into a spring in your step.[26] Her advice will also provide ample food for thought for injecting your lunchtime lull with a dose of life.

As I stated before, this book shares the stories and recommendations from various experts whose methods may differ from the Paleo/Whole30 diet I subscribe to. Yet through their stories, I share what worked for them and countless others making their journey toward a healthy, balanced life.

After winning the last battle in her war with cancer by cleansing her own body, Elissa has committed her life to helping others cleanse their toxins and to live confidently inside a healthy body. When Elissa got out of college, she wanted the fast life of a "successful" businesswoman and moved to New York City. She worked long hours at a stressful job, fueling herself with caffeine and expensive restaurant dinners. Exercise was a luxury, and sleep was for those who didn't care about moving up the ladder. She wanted to conquer the world. Then she felt a lump. When the doctor told her she had Hodgkin's lymphoma, she was stunned. She was only 32; people like her didn't get cancer. She had gotten married and was going to start a family. She had her whole life ahead of her. Now what?!

Her doctor recommended chemotherapy and radiation, but after a few treatments, she felt like the solution was worse than the problem. She realized that, in addition to medical treatment, her body needed nourishment and love. After a lot of research and listening to her inner voice, she shortened her radiation regimen and pursued an alternative path.

Elissa left her job, began managing her stress and doing yoga, and learned that what people told her was good food wasn't always *healthy* food. She began juicing and eating a more plant-based diet, and within a few months she began to heal more efficiently. Elissa and her husband, Marc, had two gorgeous daughters and cherished the life they had created together, until cancer came back into her life. But not for her. This time it was Marc's health that began to fail. Marc's doctors convinced him to begin immediate chemotherapy and radiation. He spent time in and out of hospitals as his immune system weakened. After an 18-month battle, it wasn't cancer per se that took his life; it was infection that his weakened system could not fend off. The treatment that was supposed to cure him contributed to his untimely death at 45. Elissa's run-ins with cancer showed her the importance of living a healthy, well-balanced life. After losing Marc, she went back to school at the American University of Complementary Medicine in Los Angeles and became a certified nutritionist.

Elissa really emphasizes consuming whole food, rather than packaged food. Understanding that that can be tricky for some people, Elissa recommends grabbing an apple, a banana, or some berries, as opposed to chips, crackers, or cookies. Go for something that is real food, rather than processed or packaged. Be aware of the gluten, sugar, and dairy contents. And don't feel overwhelmed if you get stuck; there are a lot of great options out there today.

The first major change Elissa recognized as a result of her new diet pertained to her energy level; second, she felt more clear-headed, and not so foggy upstairs. Finally, she noticed her sleeping patterns dramatically improved. Suddenly, it became easier to get to sleep and stay asleep, and Elissa felt that she was actually getting a restful night's sleep, which is crucial in healing and repairing the body.

Elissa makes a lot of the stuff she eats and offers some of her own easy recipes. For breakfast, she eats her own **homemade granola** with some berries and unsweetened almond or cashew milk on top. Granola contains filling sources of protein; it's a satiating snack, easy to grab, and something you can safely store in your desk at the office. **Acai berries** are a grape-like fruit packed with antioxidants, fiber, and healthy fats, benefiting your heart and digestive system.

Please refer to the Appendix, pages 192-198, for all of these great meals.

Elissa understands that more and more people are living their lives on the go, travelling to get from point A to point B, and may need the convenience of a protein bar, so she created a delicious homemade **chocolate chip protein bar** that you can stash in your briefcase, gym bag, purse, pantry, or desk drawer for easy nutrition. Each batch yields a dozen bars and will leave you with more than enough to enjoy throughout the week. With store-bought bars costing an average of $4 apiece, this is also an economical way to get in those omega- and protein-rich nuts and seeds, that energy-boosting coconut, and the sweet richness of nondairy dark chocolate. I promise you will feel satisfied and nourished throughout the day.

Another common practice for those on the go is the propensity to consume lots of coffee. But often, the caffeine crash can drain both your afternoon energy level as well as your wallet. If you prefer tea to coffee, Elissa has a recipe, although she warns that "this is not a breakfast for the faint of heart." **Elissa's matcha green tea latte** (see page 196) uses the same principle as Bulletproof Coffee but is made with antioxidant-rich green tea instead. Bulletproof Coffee is coffee with unsalted butter and a XCT oil added. In her recipe for matcha latte, she adds XCT oil or high-quality coconut oil for energy and satiation—and don't forget the butter. This breakfast treat is packed with omega-3s and vitamin D (brain fuel for the day). Perhaps the best part is that there's no coffee crash, and it's a major craving killer. The calorie count and nutrient content are meant to replace a meal, rather than to be paired with one. It's also easy to take with you to work in a travel mug, so it can stay warm as you head out the door.

A quick go-to snack that everyone should have on hand in their home and office fridge is **Elissa's homemade hummus** (see page 198). Pair this with fresh veggies or gluten-free crackers, and you will have a healthy snack full of flavor. Have fun and get creative with your recipes by adding some red pepper chili, turmeric, curry, jalapeños, or even some Kalamata olives for a Mediterranean twist.

If you want to add another fun and healthy option to your snacks or sandwiches that offers both flavor and flair, Elissa recommends an almond cheese spread that tastes like dairy cheese. It's made with almonds, is dairy-free, and provides a fantastic addition to cut-up veggies and gluten-free crackers. Try spreading some on a piece of gluten-free bread with tomato, avocado, fresh herbs, sprouts, and sea salt. You will love it!

## Develop a Dinner Routine

What's your routine for dinner? Do you find yourself thinking about what you'll have for dinner as you pull into the driveway, or did you plan ahead, knowing today would be long, and throw some things in the Crock-Pot before leaving the house? Whatever your answer may be, we could all use some help in this particularly difficult area: planning ahead.

If you work from home, cook dinner early in the day. Cook after breakfast before the slump hits and while the kitchen is still a mess and dishes are dirty. Never wait until 5 p.m. to start cooking if you have afternoon slumps. If you work outside the home, use planned leftovers, or try one of the hundreds of healthy, delicious, easy meals out there that require little effort other than throwing some meat, fresh herbs, and veggies into the Crock-Pot and pressing the start button before you leave the house. To help get you started, I've set you up with my easy **Laurie's Crock-Pot Chicken Enchilada Stew** recipe (see page 198) that will cook itself while you're at work and is a great meal for when it's cold outside. I also love serving this as an alternative to chili during football season because of how healthy and satisfying it leaves you.

Try and cook on the weekends or batch cook in the evenings and stock the freezer with the parts and pieces or full meals you need in order to get dinner on the table fast. Make a list and don't forget to thaw things by popping the already cooked pieces in the fridge the night before so they're easier to deal with once you get home from work. If you have a good day, fix extras in case you have a bad day tomorrow. Chopped veggies will keep a few days in the fridge, no problem, and some will also freeze well depending on the item. If you find yourself in a jam, double the meal and eat the leftovers the next night.

If you work from home and have enough energy in the afternoon, do your prep work ahead of time. Chop the veggies in advance and store them in the fridge. Make any needed sauces or sides and put them all in resealable containers to use throughout the week.

If you work outside the home, prepping ahead can be a major advantage to getting dinner on the table faster. Chop all the veggies and make all the sauces you'll need for the week on the weekend. I also like to portion the veggies into separate containers and freeze them if necessary. I also recommend roasting chickens on Sundays and freezing the leftover meat.

My last piece of advice is to always have a backup plan. Always keep a meal in the freezer in case things go south and you have to choose between a freezer meal and calling for delivery. Always assume there will be days when you'll have to stay late at the office, forget to stop by the market on the way home, pick your kid up late from practice, etc. It's critical to keep your freezer stocked for those days. And remember that a meal with nonorganic, butter-cooked veggies or grocery store meat is better than fast food or a pizza, so don't kill yourself with grief if you get stuck.

As you prepare for dinner and lunch this week, try a terrific **Summer Vegetable Minestrone** soup recipe from Elissa (see pages 199-200) that will boost your serotonin and help heal depression. The amino acids L-tryptophan and L-tyrosine are building blocks for the neurotransmitter serotonin and the catecholamine hormones (basically your stress hormones involved in the fight-or-flight responses). Making sure that you have plenty of these in your diet from quality lean meat such as turkey or chicken, avocados, and seeds can really support your tolerance of stress as well as your mental well-being. I also recommend my own Paleo/ Whole30 **Panang Curry Chicken/Shrimp** (see pages 200-201) and **Light and Spicy Baked Coconut Fish** (see page 201). Both can be made in under an hour after getting home from the office, and both are extremely healthy and delicious.

Exercise, healthy food, rest, and relaxation will help you to develop and maintain your emotional and mental strength. By taking good care of yourself, you are sending your brain signals that you deserve to be taken care of. Make sure you are devoting as much time as possible to meeting your basic needs for food, exercise, sleep, and relaxation. As you work through making these important changes, small and large, constantly repeat the following to yourself: "I am worth living. I'm worth living, and I'm worth having a great life. I'm worth eating good and healthy food, and I'm worth the extra time necessary to be good to my body." Finally, consider the following question: Junk food you've craved for an hour, or the body you've craved for a lifetime?

Now, how would you answer?

# CHAPTER 4

# SLEEP IS NOT FOR THE WEAK

Four to five hours, max. That was my average sleep time during the 2008 presidential campaign to elect then-Senator Barack Obama. I was managing the political operation for the state of Florida, and I had eight guys reporting to me, each located in a different part of the state. The work was super stressful. All around the world, people were watching to see "if Florida would *eff up* the election again," and a large part of my job entailed making sure the elected officials and surrogates (celebrities, local and national politicians, dignitaries, etc.) were kept happy. We needed all of these people to help gin up the base, increasing voter turnout come election day. After all, the world was watching to see if the Sunshine State would have another election outcome like in 2000 with Gore vs. Bush.

The job was great, don't get me wrong. I had wonderful people working for me, most of whom joined me afterwards to work in the Administration. Yet on an individual basis, it wasn't always easy during that time. We all struggled in our own way, and as a result, many of us ended up consuming shitty food, going out every night drinking, chain-smoking, enduring a constant caffeine overload, or hooking up with coworkers just to feel a temporary connection with a person while living through the highs and lows of the campaign. Some people were able to hold it together, but for most, this was everyday life as a staffer. Surprisingly, there were a number of couples who met while working on the campaign in one of the various battleground states, and a few even got hitched. But that was definitely not the norm among various social circles.

My colleagues and I would frequently go out drinking after work to let off steam and continue "team building," as we liked to call it. In truth, most days ran around fourteen hours, which only got increasingly worse after August and through Election Day, so we felt we didn't really need an excuse to "drown one's sorrows" and gorge on the bar food that came along with it. The problem was, we carried on with that pattern almost every night through November. I began telling myself that if I just kept moving and didn't stop, I could keep going all night and still wake up in the morning to do it all over again. I finally took a pause when I fell asleep at the wheel while waiting in line to pay a toll after dropping off actress Cynthia Nixon at the airport. The attendant had been tapping on my window, telling me I needed to pay when I came to.

Furious with myself because I knew better, I pulled over at the next exit, slept for about an hour in a parking lot, and then continued making my way across the state, daydreaming of my bed and how badly I wanted to rest my eyes. I was taken by surprise from the numbing pain in my legs and neck. I was exhausted and depleted not just physically, but mentally, as well. Why didn't I do anything to fix this terrible state in which I'd found myself? All the signs were there, staring me in the face, yet I continued to push, turning those red flags green.

I think we all realize that sleep makes us feel better, but its importance goes way beyond just boosting our mood or banishing under-eye circles. Sleep is essential for a person's health and well-being, according to the National Sleep Foundation (NSF). Yet millions of people do not get enough sleep, and many suffer from a lack of sleep. In 2014, the NSF conducted its first ever population-level poll—The 2014 Sleep Index™—to track the nation's changing sleep habits, problems, behaviors, and beliefs. Most of the findings were not surprising but clearly demonstrated that Americans need to do better between the sheets and get more sleep.[27]

Most individuals suffer the occasional sleepless night or periods of poor sleep during stressful life events such as a job or home struggle, an illness, the birth of a child, a marriage, or a death. For many people, the occasional sleep problems can evolve into chronic insomnia. The NSF's 2014 Sleep Index™ found that only 35 percent of Americans reported their sleep quality as "good" and 23 percent as "only fair." African Americans were more likely to report poor or failing sleep quality than non-Hispanic whites. Seventeen percent of respondents had been told by a physician that they have a sleep disorder, and only 18 percent of individuals said they would choose sleep if they had an extra hour in the day.

For most people, these problems go undiagnosed and untreated and can quickly lead to a serious problem. Fortunately, there has been a significant amount of research devoted to sleep and insomnia that has uncovered many things you can do to improve your sleep. With more and more people suffering from the side effects of sleep medications, cognitive behavioral therapy (CBT-I) is now recommended to be the first-line treatment for adults with chronic insomnia by the American College of Physicians.[28]

Ronald Kotler, MD, DABSM, Medical Director at the Pennsylvania Hospital Sleep Disorders Center, stated that in the early 1900s, the average adult got about nine hours of sleep.[29] In the year 2000, the average adult got about seven hours of sleep, and that average has remained basically the same today. The NSF found that the average bedtime on weekdays for the American population is 10:55 p.m., with a 6:38 a.m. wake-up time. So, the key question at hand is, why are we getting less sleep? Do we need less sleep today than we did a century ago? Kotler says the answer is "no!" Nevertheless, the fact is that we are getting less sleep. If we go back to our ancestors who worked on the farm, we come to realize that our sleep schedule was dependent upon how light it was outside. If it was nighttime and dark, people slept. Conversely, when it was light out, people worked. Everything changed after Thomas Edison invented the light bulb, which gave us the ability to stay awake at any time of day.

With the use of artificial lights and stimulants such as caffeine, we are able to fight off the physiological need to sleep. The danger is that we need sleep to feel refreshed, for hormonal balance, for physical and mental repair, and for memory consolidation. According to Kotler, when we don't get enough sleep, we take away our ability to undergo a very important process that allows our bodies to heal and feel refreshed, increasing the chance for long-term consequences.

The average adult needs seven to nine hours of sleep, and it is biologically determined for each individual so that different people need different amounts of sleep within that range. However, according to Kotler, people who say they can get by on less sleep are often masking a physiological tendency toward sleep, often by staying very active. For example, Kotler recalls the time when he was a medical intern starved of sleep and the only way he could stay awake was to remain active. He just kept moving, going from patient room to patient room, but the moment he sat down for a lecture, it became easy for him to fall asleep. By playing these games, not only do we rob ourselves of the need to get restored and refreshed, but also, Kotler says that it can also contribute to medical disorders and premature death.

Furthermore, Kotler warns that if we are sleep-deprived, it is going to be more of a challenge to deal with the daily stresses of life. For example, for those who have children, you know that when they're very young, they can disrupt your sleep, which can affect a person's mood and tolerance level for problem solving and just makes the person cranky in general. This stress can contribute to depression, anger, and arguments, so it makes sense to deal with life's stresses in a rational way. One of the most important ways to combat stress is to get a good night's sleep so you have the tools, emotionally and intellectually, to deal with such stresses.

## Road Warriors

Do you travel for work and feel like you live out of your suitcase? I've lived like that for most of my career, allowing my job to dictate my personal schedule, sleep time, meals, etc. It became unbearable when I began travelling between different time zones, which made it impossible to get a peaceful night's sleep.

Dr. Kotler offers recommendations for people who travel to the same city multiple times that they try to reproduce the same environment by bringing things from home, whether it's a pillow, pictures, or scents like lavender linen spray. Try staying in the same hotel, and even go so far as requesting the same room. Make sure your room is away from the elevator on a floor that's high enough so you won't hear ground-level noise, and make sure you bring your workout gear. Kotler says it should be a priority to work out whenever you're on the road. If you know your hotel has a fitness center and/or a swimming pool, be sure to throw the proper gear in your suitcase. You'll feel better if you do so.

It's also important to eat sensibly on the road. Sometimes when people travel, they overdo it and go out to restaurants, eat more food than they should (and perhaps drink more alcohol than they should), and eat later than they should. Well, here's the truth: all of those things mentioned are going to disrupt your sleep. So try and keep those similar habits, similar bed times, similar meal times, etc. And if you have an important meeting that may keep you up late, in fear that you won't wake up, Dr. Kotler recommends setting a couple of alarm clocks. Set your own alarm clock and also ask the front desk to schedule a wake-up call. That way you have a backup that you can rely on.

For Bill Nye, the key to his success when he's on the road is sleep. "You gotta sleep people. You have to sleep," he says. He claims that he learned to nap early on, during his years of standup comedy attempts, and became quite good at napping, in fact. Bill's preferred nap time is twenty-two minutes but says sometimes you have to take what you can get. Whether it's twenty-two minutes or seven, Bill says some time is better than no time, and "sometimes you gotta do what you gotta do." To relax, Bill enjoys reading ("yes, actual books," he says. He's currently reading *The Serengeti Rules: The Quest to Discover How Life Works and Why It Matters* by Sean B. Carroll) and says that reading may be helpful for people having trouble falling asleep.

## The Dos and the Dims

*"The worst thing in the world is to try to sleep and not to."*
—F. Scott Fitzgerald

What is insomnia? We hear about it, but what exactly are the two major classes of sleep disorders? Dr. Kotler says there are the dos and the dims. The dos are the disorders of excessive sleepiness such as sleep apnea and narcolepsy. The dims are the disorders of initiating and maintaining sleep. Kotler says that insomnia is a disorder of initiating and maintaining sleep but isn't considered a disorder unless it begins to bother the patient. A lot of patients have difficulty falling asleep or staying asleep, but it doesn't particularly bother them. It becomes labeled a disorder when it becomes a problem for the patient, who is unhappy with the fact that he/she doesn't sleep well. It can, in turn, affect his/her daytime functioning, and he/she can feel tired during the day. A lot of times this will affect a person who has a predisposition, or a precipitating factor such as a negative life event, like a divorce, the death of a family member, or the loss of a job.

Even a positive event like getting married can affect your sleep because anything that is stimulating to the brain will interfere with your ability to fall asleep and stay asleep.

Dr. Kotler offers advice on how to deal with insomnia: he says there are a number of factors that promote good overall sleep hygiene. For example, going to bed at the same time every night, getting up at the same time every morning, allowing yourself eight hours of sleep, and avoiding staying in bed for more than thirty minutes if you can't fall asleep (or you can't get back to sleep) all contribute. If you wake up and you can't get back to sleep within thirty minutes, Kotler suggests getting out of bed and going to a quiet spot in your house. It is important that you not stay in bed awake for long periods of time because you will eventually start to associate the bed with a place where you don't sleep and then it self-perpetuates. Once you've relocated from your bed, find a comfortable chair with a dim light and no electronic devices (light tells the brain that it's time to be awake). Sit quietly with a dim light and read until you feel tired and can go back into the bedroom.

Of course, what you eat and drink prior to trying to fall asleep can also impact your ability to successfully get to bed in time. You need to recognize that there are things like caffeine, alcohol, and tobacco products that are very bad for sleep. Nutritionist Elissa Goodman suggests drinking tart cherry juice if you're having trouble sleeping.[30] Cherries are one of only a few natural foods that contain melatonin, the chemical from the pineal gland in the brain that helps control the body's internal clock. Elissa also suggests gluten-free carbs at dinner because they can calm down the central nervous system. Try gluten-free grains, chick peas, sweet potatoes, leafy greens, and kale. One of Elissa's favorite foods before bed is a banana, which helps promote sleep because of the magnesium and potassium that act as natural muscle relaxants. Elissa says she also takes a magnesium supplement every night before bed because it acts as a sleep booster, and getting the proper minerals into the body daily is essential. Minerals regulate your metabolism and are crucial for your health and well-being. The existence of proper minerals in your body can even improve your workouts if you exercise regularly.

Dr. Kotler says that exercise promotes healthy sleep and it can also increase endorphins and serotonin and other good chemicals that make you feel good and help you deal with stress. Kotler believes that most people who have stressful lives will tell you that after an aerobic workout, they see things differently and are able to deal with the stresses of life and decision making more easily, which will allow less mind racing when you try to fall asleep.

I agree with Dr. Kotler 100 percent! If I have learned anything from CrossFit, it's that every time I put myself through a grueling workout, my body and my mind get stronger and allow me to do the things I once thought were impossible. There's this saying I've heard a lot of coaches yell out (putting their own spin on it) to their athletes as they leave the gym after finishing a workout: "this is the hardest thing you'll do all day; the rest is easy." It took me about a month of going four to five days a week at six o'clock in the morning to really get it. Having to get up at five o'clock in the morning to make a six a.m. class so I could still get to work on time sucked, because it also meant I had to get to bed earlier the night before. But I quickly realized that by the time class was over, I had already done so much hard work, and it was only seven o'clock. I didn't hit snooze on my alarm. I got my ass to the gym and moved through pain, fatigue, stress, and exhaustion and came out stronger sixty minutes later. My confidence eventually grew (shit, I just deadlifted 135 lbs), and I began to approach every day as if there were nothing anyone could throw at me that I couldn't handle. My new morning motto became "bring it on!"

Dr. Kotler says that someone who has insomnia is more likely to get better if they are part of an aerobic exercise program. If you are having trouble getting good sleep, exercise (assuming it's not too close to bedtime) is great because it causes biochemical changes in the brain that promote good, healthy sleep. According to the National Sleep Foundation, "People sleep significantly better and feel more alert during the day if they get at least 150 minutes of exercise a week. A nationally representative sample of more than 2,600 men and women, ages 18-85, found that 150 minutes of moderate to vigorous activity a week, which is the national guideline, provided a 65 percent improvement in sleep quality. People also said they felt less sleepy during the day, compared to those with less physical activity."[31]

## Up, All Night

While working at the White House, Phil Larson admitted to sleeping in his office more than a few times. Whether he was working on the Fukushima nuclear disaster in Japan after the earthquake or the gulf oil spill off the coast of Louisiana, launching a new initiative, or getting a new government website up and running, Phil was working around the clock. As a result, sleeping in the office sometimes became necessary. Unfortunately for Phil, worrying about everyone and everything besides himself made it difficult to fall asleep most nights, triggering symptoms of fatigue, irritability, and forgetfulness. It has been said that the metabolism of a White House is set by its occupant, so if Barack Obama is a night owl, then it's not a surprise that long nights and weekend meetings were business as usual. I mean, we are talking about working for the president of the United States. But, still, who here thinks someone will be at their best after sleeping on a couch for a few hours?

Dr. Kotler said, and the American College of Physicians agrees,[32] that the most important current treatment for insomnia is cognitive behavioral therapy, as opposed to over-the-counter or prescription medicines on which people used to rely. In Dr. Kotler's sleep program at the Pennsylvania Hospital Sleep Disorder Center, they have nurse practitioners who are trained to give cognitive behavioral therapy for those suffering from sleep disorders, using behavioral interventions such as sleep restriction, stimulus control, and educating the patient on sleep hygiene (for example, if a patient is struggling with the fact that he/she lies in bed for eight hours but only sleeps six hours). To address this, a sleep restriction approach would be to have the patient stay in bed for only six hours until their sleep efficiency increases. A nurse or a psychologist administering cognitive behavioral therapy would then gradually increase the amount of time in the bed so the patient receives more sleep.

It is important for a patient to start off by giving a detailed history about their sleep, sleep patterns, when they started having trouble, what was the precipitant to when they started losing sleep, and whether they are taking medicines that might interfere with sleep or using tobacco, alcohol, nicotine products, or stimulants. It's also important that the patient keep an extensive sleep diary that accounts for all of their sleep habits. Once this has been done, the cognitive behavioral therapist will go over some of the things that may be interfering with the patient's sleep and will review the sleep hygiene and sleep restrictions, also identifying any distorted thinking.

By identifying distorted or negative thinking, Kotler says you can then entice the patient with more rational interpretations of events that play a large role in sleep. An example would be a patient who lies in bed and can't fall asleep and starts to assume (due to distorted thinking) that if they don't sleep, something bad is going to happen—e.g., they will lose their job and have big problems. Distorted thinking is also known as cognitive distortion, which is a big part of depression and insomnia, and Kotler says the two go hand in hand. Particularly for patients who have insomnia, anxiety, depression, or a combination of the three, those things would need to be addressed.

Dr. Kotler uses cognitive behavioral therapy as part of his eight-session program. There is one weekly session, with the first session lasting an hour, and subsequently seven thirty-minute sessions over the course of eight weeks, which can lead to substantial benefits. Kotler recommends alternative options that have been shown to improve sleep such as yoga, meditation, and relaxation techniques.

Dr. Kotler says there's a part of the brain called the suprachiasmatic nucleus (SCN), located in the hypothalamus, which generates our circadian rhythms ("circa" meaning "around," and "dies" meaning the day). As referenced in *ScienceDaily*, "A circadian rhythm is a roughly 24-hour cycle in the physiological processes of living beings. In a strict sense, circadian rhythms are endogenously generated, although they can be modulated by external cues such as sunlight and temperature."[33] Kotler explains that these rhythms are a type of biorhythm, and there are many biorhythms in the body such as hormone production like cortisol. One circadian rhythm is the sleep/awake cycle. The neuronal and hormonal activities generated regulate many different body functions in a 24-hour cycle, using around 20,000 neurons.

Kotler says there are people who have what is known as Delayed Sleep Phase Syndrome (DSPS), where their biorhythm is to go to bed at 3 a.m. and get up at 11 a.m. He also says he has patients who come in with a particular biorhythm. For example, an actor who goes to bed late at night and gets up late in the morning might have developed a unique biorhythm. Kotler says this can become a problem when a person tries to conform to conventional society and has to work a job that's not in sync with their circadian rhythm.

DSPS was first seen in people during their teenage years, or adolescence. Kotler says it's very common for teenagers to want to stay up really late and get up really late. Many people argue that, by starting school too early, teenagers end up being less productive because their schedule is out of sync with their circadian rhythms. Many people argue that it would be much better to start school later and end later so that it is more in sync with the typical circadian rhythm of a teenager. It becomes a problem when the teenagers can't adjust to a typical work schedule that requires them to rise and shine (as well as fall asleep) at more conventional times. For example, someone who has DSPS can go to college, pick all late classes, and be quite successful for four years—perhaps with a 3 a.m. bedtime and an 11 a.m. wake-up time. Then, when the student graduates Phi Beta Kappa, gets a great job on Wall Street, and their boss says to them, "Okay, I'll see you at 7:30 in the morning," they freak out when they can't get to sleep that night. That person now has a big problem, and that's what Kotler says is referred to as DSPS.

Austin Willard, cadet at West Point, knows all too well about sleep deprivation. Sure, Austin's a college student, and like most of his peers, he stays up late studying; but for Austin, he doesn't have the luxury of creating his own schedule where he can choose to have his earliest class be at eleven o'clock in the morning, for example. Austin, who studies and works on homework until almost one a.m. every night, often finds it hard to get up in the morning, so he does his workouts immediately following classes late in the afternoon. Dinner is whatever the staff brings to the table, served in the mess hall, and enjoyed with 4,600 of his closest friends. Austin tries to avoid falling into the trap of shoving Skittles and M&Ms into his mouth at all hours of the night like his roommates do, and instead he chooses to snack on healthy foods like almonds and dried fruit. He cares a lot about what he puts into his body, and if the dinner being served is just too terrible on a given evening, he and a few friends will usually cook salmon and rice for themselves in their rooms with a slow cooker or Crock-Pot. Austin says the barrack-made meals aren't always the tastiest, but they are often healthier than what the mess has to offer.

Certainly the unhealthiest thing Austin sees his fellow cadets do more so than eating involves the amount of caffeine they consume. He says he has friends who will wake up, crack open a Monster energy drink, chug the entire thing just to stay awake, go to the mess hall for breakfast, throw down several cups of coffee, and then go to class. Austin says that by the time they reach their ten o'clock class, they will go and grab another energy drink (Red Bull or Monster) to make it through the rest of the morning and then head to lunch. If the cadet can fall asleep, he/she will attempt to take a brief nap after lunch, and then on the way to his/her afternoon class, the cadet will grab another Monster drink to get through the afternoon class without falling asleep. Then after class and before he/she heads to the gym, he/she will take a preworkout supplement like C4, which is riddled with caffeine and other unhealthy ingredients, and then finally the cadet goes back to his/her barracks to study until two a.m., consuming yet another energy drink or two along the way. Austin says this is a daily ritual for most of his classmates.

Having guest-lectured at West Point myself on a few occasions, I admit I was not at all surprised by Austin's account of his peers' unhealthy habits to stay awake. As I greeted each cadet walking through the door, I couldn't help but notice a majority of them quickly consuming the remaining contents of either a black and green or silver can and chucking it into a trash bin, which had quickly filled with empty energy drink containers. I was extremely troubled at seeing this, which begged the question as to how some of our best and brightest are getting an education, hopped up on astronomical levels of caffeine. According to my calculation, if a cadet consumes a minimum of four energy drinks a day, that's a caffeine jolt equivalent of eighteen 12-oz cans of Coca-Cola. Say what?! This unhealthy habit could become extremely dangerous and addictive over time if the person continues consuming that amount of caffeine so close to bedtime, missing the required amount of sleep needed to repair the body.

Austin says it's tough to go into the field for training where you're required to eat MRE's (meals ready to eat), which is just processed food, come back to school, and immediately try to purge the body of whatever food he abused it with for two weeks. Austin swears by green tea to help detoxify his body, and lots of sleep when returning from training in the field. He says it's tough to get sleep at the Academy, even for the ones who really try, but he thinks he does pretty well, getting an average of six hours of sleep a night. Unfortunately, the same cannot be said for most of his peers, who likely get an average of four to five hours of sleep and are suffering because of it.

Austin is aware that his six hours of sleep are on the high end among most cadets, but only because he made it a priority to protect his sleep was he able to avoid other people invading it. Whether it is his fiancée or his parents back at home in Colorado who want to keep in touch but live in different time zones, Austin had to set boundaries and clear expectations with them early on regarding how they maintain contact and when they call, so it wouldn't eat into his sleep. Austin says the same can be said for the civilian world—it's all about good time management. You have to schedule your sleep time and create hard deadlines with yourself. For Austin, one o'clock in the morning is his hard stop, and anything that still has to be done will get done the following day and be done better if he is well rested.

## Flipping the switch

In 2011, having just graduated from nursing school, 2016 CrossFit Games competitor Christy Adkins began doing twelve-hour shift work (which frequently turned into thirteen-hour shifts) at a hospital. Christy had to work day shifts for two weeks and then work night shifts for two weeks, alternating back and forth. Christy says that was the worst she has ever felt performance- and training-wise. After trying to make it work for nine months, she started looking for other nursing jobs. Christy was fortunate to find a nursing job at a local ballet school in DC that fit in great with her training schedule, so she made the switch.

Dr. Kotler says that he sees patients who have crazy schedules similar to Christy's that cause the patient to feel like they constantly have jet lag because their biorhythm is unbalanced. Kotler refers to this condition as SWSD (Shift Work Sleep Disorder), and for many people this can be unsustainable. Most of Dr. Kotler's patients who have SWSD are in the field of nursing, law enforcement, public safety, etc., because we're a twenty-four-hour society. Shift work is a difficult thing to deal with because it can cause you to constantly be out of sync with your biorhythms and circadian rhythms. SWSD can cause a person to feel lousy, tired, and irritable and to endure frequent headaches. Dr. Kotler says there are some things you can do to feel a little better, but it comes down to this—if SWSD is really upsetting your life, the best thing to do is find new work. If that's not possible, you want to try and work it out with your employer that you do the same shift, and avoid rotating shifts. If you're a shift worker, try and keep that same schedule seven days a week. For example, if you're working the night shift four days a week, and three days during that week you sleep conventional hours, that is not going to be sustainable, according to Kotler.

Christy offers recommendations for folks who work similar jobs or do shift work and are struggling with poor eating habits and ever-changing sleep patterns. You have to plan your meals and make sure that you're hydrated enough and not eating sugar and junk throughout your shift. It really comes down to preplanning, which Christy says doesn't have to include an entire week, but simply having breakfast before you leave the house, even if it's super early in the morning, will make a huge difference. Regardless of how early you have to wake up for work, it is important to give yourself enough time to enjoy a good breakfast. Also, you should prepare a lunch and/or dinner for that day's shift, so there is no excuse to hit up the cafeteria or lunch truck. You already know you're going to be there for those two meals, so plan accordingly. No excuses!

Dr. Kotler will tell you there is no good remedy to constantly switching shifts because your biorhythm is constantly out of balance, and as you get older it gets harder to sustain. There are some things you can do to help. For example, if you're working the night shift, wear sunglasses on the way home, limiting your exposure to bright light since you're going to want to fall asleep as soon as you get home. Kotler also recommends making sure your bedroom is quiet and the phone is turned off. Don't be afraid to have a friendly chat with your neighbor if they happen to mow their lawn early Saturday or Sunday mornings. Most people will understand once you explain. It is essential to have a quiet, darkened room and sleep the same hours every day. Unfortunately, Kotler says there's no good answer to the disruption caused by constantly changing shifts and advises his patients if at all possible, when they come in feeling lousy because they are having rotating shifts, to try and find a job where they can work the same shift, even if it's the night shift. Sometimes that can be done by keeping the same profession, like in Christy's case, and sometimes you have to change professions. But Kotler explains that there are no easy solutions for someone experiencing lots of problems with constantly changing shifts.

Dr. Kotler says that in life, each of us has our own set of priorities. If you have a partner, he or she should be on the same wavelength and share your priorities, or it won't work. For Kotler, his top priority in life is wellness, and he just happened to learn at an early age what it takes to feel well—

sleep. Kotler is rigid about his own sleep and also about the amount of exercise he gets. He is fortunate to have an understanding spouse who knows his emotional well-being is dependent on his getting good sleep, exercising, eating well, keeping a sound mind, and maintaining a balanced life to the extent that he can as a doctor. Sometimes it can be as simple as making the decision that these things are important to you.

Kotler says he has patients with poor sleep habits who come in seeking help, but it's not necessarily their top priority, and therefore they have trouble achieving their desired result. Some of Kotler's patients are poor, working multiple jobs, or are single parents working multiple jobs while also taking care of multiple kids or an aging parent. Just remember that it may be easy for us to sit and talk about how important it is to get good sleep and exercise, but the reality is, for some people to make a living it's very hard, and their priorities are different. For many people, their priority is putting food on the table. So for those who have the luxury of getting the recommended seven to eight hours of sleep, and going to the gym several times a week, you have to make the decision for your own health and well-being that it's going to be a priority.

My hope is that most of you have already "decided" that being well is a priority. You want to feel well, which in turn makes you feel happy, right? Being healthy means taking care of your body by getting good sleep, exercising, and eating well, all of which are top priorities. If you give yourself a few weeks to master each set of the self-help techniques given throughout this chapter and practice them regularly, your sleep should improve significantly. Don't be so hard on yourself if you come up against the occasional sleepless night, and remember that even good sleepers have nights of poor sleep. It may not always be easy, but by adopting these techniques as a part of your permanent daily behavior, you are on your way to improved sleep and relaxation.

# CHAPTER 5

# CHILL OUT AND TAKE A MOMENT TO BREATHE

During the 2012 presidential campaign, I was sitting at my desk, earbuds in, listening to Drake's "The Motto," when suddenly the office bully came tearing out of his office like a tiger, running over to my desk, eyes bugged out, hands flailing, and yelling something that I couldn't hear because my music was still blaring in my ears. Feeling the hairs on my arms and legs stick up, I slowly turned my swivel office chair around and tried not to remain within distance of the spit that was coming out of his mouth every time he spoke. I pulled out one ear bud, took a deep breath, and said, "Can I help you with something?"

That seemed to have made him even angrier—now he was really freaking out and swinging his arms back and forth while screaming at the top of his lungs. It was impressive, really, the level of intensity that he was able to keep up while getting absolutely no feedback from me.

While he was screaming, I was doing a form of meditation. By closing my eyes and focusing on mentally blocking out his noise, I was able to let go of everything happening around me, focusing instead on the music playing in my ears and visualizing what I was going to cook for dinner that night.

I thought about all of the ingredients I was going to add to my salad. I debated whether I should grill or bake the fish I had taken out of the freezer that morning, and whether or not I had enough spinach and tomatoes left in the fridge.

It's not like I'm a monk or anything. I started practicing mindfulness after the 2008 campaign because I was looking for a way to control and release stress in a healthy way, rather than via late-night binge drinking or eating "comfort" food that was terribly bad for me. I had been running to relieve the stress, but it really wasn't leaving me feeling fully satisfied— only more tired and restless. Then I was introduced to meditation through yoga. Meditation involves an internal effort to self-regulate, calming the mind, reducing stress and anxiety, gathering energy to overcome exhaustion, and balancing mind, body, and spirit. While meditation is not a religion or a philosophy, it paves the way to inner peace and pays respect to the ultimate source of all human accomplishment.

Meditation can literally change our brains, improving our capacity for decision making, and enhance our emotional intelligence and our ability to act with clarity and wisdom, alone and in concert with others. All I needed that day was for my meditation to stop me from ripping out the guy's throat and reacting to his ridiculous behavior.

I'm glad that some well-timed meditation allowed me to stay strong and not justify the office bully's behavior with a response. I had also hoped the staff, especially the younger ones that he picked on all the time, got the message that inappropriate behavior would not be tolerated and go unnoticed, even in the "wild west" of a presidential campaign.

## Mind Full, or Mindful?

Oprah Winfrey, one of the most powerful women in the world, trains hard to keep herself physically healthy. In an interview with *O Magazine*, Winfrey said her workouts include "45 minutes of cardio six mornings a week, four to five strength-training sessions a week, incline crunches, and stretching." Winfrey also admits to sitting in silence for 20 minutes, twice a day. Oprah said transcendental meditation (TM) leaves her feeling "full of hope, a sense of contentment, and joy knowing for sure that even in the daily craziness that bombards us from every direction, there is—still—the constancy of stillness." Oprah even brought in TM teachers who taught everyone in her company who wanted to learn how to meditate. "The results were awesome and they reported sleeping better, having improved relationships with spouses, partners, children, and co-workers."[34]

Congressman Tim Ryan of Ohio, author of *A Mindful Nation* and *The Real Food Revolution*, discovered meditation while looking for a way to reduce stress. Finding meditation was life-changing for him, and he embarked on a campaign to bring the benefits of mindfulness to government and education.

Ryan, on a quest to make America more zen, is also a yogi and understands the benefits of mental and physical wellness, particularly in how we treat our veterans. He brought yoga to Capitol Hill by sponsoring "Yoga on the Hill," which has since become an annual event raising awareness of mental health and suicide prevention. I was fortunate to have participated in both these forums. It was truly spectacular to be a part of a yoga session held inside the capitol, open to everyone, with participants that included members of Congress, their staff, and veterans.

## Warrior at Ease

Through Ryan, I met Dan Nevins, wounded warrior and yoga instructor. Despite Dan's near-death experience and the loss of both legs, he approaches life with an emotional strength that makes him an ideal example of how to mentally adapt to a challenging situation.[35]

Nevins, then a Staff Sergeant, recalled the exact hour that his life changed forever—it was four o'clock in the morning on November 10, 2004, in Balad, Iraq, and he and his squadron were headed out on what was supposed to be a seventy-two-hour dismounted counterinsurgent operation. Having learned that their base, LSA Anaconda, Balad Air Base, was going to be attacked, they decided through their battle plan that they would meet the enemy where they were, eliminating the threat of coordinated assaults.

It was pitch-black outside, and his squadron was driving down a pitiful dirt road, not even a kilometer from their base and onto what was intended to be their dismounted site. Dan, with his head down, was praying for safety, wisdom, and the ability to make tactical decisions when he suddenly heard a *boom*. A roadside bomb had detonated near their vehicle.

The silence destroyed by the deafening blast sent Dan's vehicle, weighing 18,000 pounds, six feet in the air in a ball of fire. With his head bowed in a prayer position, all Dan remem-bers is hearing and feeling the Humvee basically disintegrate around his body. Having been knocked unconscious at some point, Dan opened his eyes, realizing he had been ejected from his vehicle. Now lying in the soft dirt, still covered in darkness, with only a faint light from the lingering fire from the blast, Dan saw that his legs were still caught in the twisted and burning metal of what used to be the floorboard and undercarriage of the truck. As the dust descended around Dan, he noticed his weapon lying nearby on the ground, and his inner "soldier" immediately kicked in. "Dan, get up, sit up, put your weapon in operation," he told himself, not knowing what could happen next. After many attempts to sit up, he realized he physically couldn't and instead lay back against the vehicle. He looked over toward the driver's compartment and saw that his good friend, Staff Sgt. Michael Ottolini, had been killed, making the ultimate sacrifice.

Not really understanding the extent of his own injuries, through blurred eyes Dan remembers feeling proud as he watched his team doing everything they were supposed to do to keep the area safe, moving into tactical proficiency. During all of the chaos around him, Dan remembers trying to hear the noise that usually came following an ambush (air raid sirens, the thump of shellfire, the roar of rockets). Not hearing any, he thought, *okay, I have some time* and began checking himself out. He started with his head, and his helmet came apart in a couple of pieces in his hand. He knew that wasn't a good start. He then began to check his torso, reaching up for his legs since he was still on the ground with his legs inside the vehicle. When he went to reach up for them, he felt the unmistakable arterial blood spurt through his hand. That was when Dan realized he was going to die. With everything starting to slow down, as he lay there basically giving up, he started to make his peace with God and say good-bye to his wife and daughter.

Dan thought he was done. But then, a strange thing happened: instead of Dan's life flashing before his eyes, his experience was just the opposite. Dan began to have flashes of all of the things he hadn't yet done. The one that really got to Dan—the one flash that really zapped him awake— was watching his daughter walk down the aisle with no father to give her away on her wedding day. With this, Dan suddenly woke up. This time he told himself, "Dan, you're alive. You're alive, do something!" So Dan stuck his hand into his wound, trying to find the artery, and pressed down hard, praying that he could slow the bleeding enough until a medic arrived.

In what seemed like the blink of an eye, he suddenly found that a medic was putting a tourniquet on his leg. He blinked and saw his team leader putting an IV in his arm, and blinking again he saw his entire team there, putting themselves in harm's way to free and release what remained of his legs from the truck that was still on fire. In another blink, Dan was placed on a stretcher, then a helicopter, and then on his way to a surgical hospital. He remembers waking up from that surgery in the hospital in Balad, Iraq, and seeing a nurse's face right in front of his. He has never forgotten her face and never knew her name, but she said something to Dan that he will never forget: "Sgt. Nevins, you're a very lucky man. We managed to repair your femoral artery and had to give you a lot of blood. We had to take your left leg below the knee. We managed to save most of your right one for now—but you'll probably lose that one too."

The nurse was right. Three years later, after spending almost two years at Walter Reed Army Medical Center in Washington, DC, and going through more than thirty surgeries, they took his right leg as well.

Having been transported to LRMC (Landstuhl Regional Medical Center) in Germany, Dan remembers feeling sorry for himself. The whole time Dan stayed there, all he could think of was what that nurse said to him, which was that he lost his leg and would probably lose the other one as well. Dan asked himself, "What can a guy with no legs do?" In his mind, the answer was "nothing." Dan had always defined himself by his physical achievements: he was a competitive runner, and running was what had brought him and his wife together, sharing that same passion. It's what they did, it was part of how they met, and now that was gone. "Would she love me anymore?" Dan questioned. And then he began to think about his daughter and how he would put her up on his shoulders and run around. He thought of how his daughter looked up to him and respected him for his strength. Now he questioned how she would even do that anymore. Dan spent the next seven days setting himself up for a lifetime of disappointment and loneliness.

Once he was at Walter Reed, there was only one person Dan felt he could talk to and trust—his nurse, Erica. That is, until he was introduced to some folks from the Wounded Warrior Project. Dan says the members of the WWP changed his life, introducing him to sports and for the first time showing him that his disability didn't have to define him, that he himself could define what his life was going to be like. The WWP staff was there for Dan throughout his entire stay at

Walter Reed and thirty-some-odd surgeries. The organization provided Dan with opportunities to snowboard, wakeboard, etc., and he learned to heal from his physical wounds of war pretty quickly. At the same time, by thrusting himself into the world of this adrenaline rush that accompanied beating people, it brought on a competitive ego for Dan, something that he had not felt in some time.

Dan learned to use his prosthetics pretty well thanks to Laura Friedman, a really great physical therapist at Walter Reed who gave him guidance on how to walk and become pretty good on two prosthetic legs very quickly.

Nevertheless, the attempt to go back to daily life as he knew it before the war was not easy. Dan initially went back to working at Pfizer as a drug rep, but ultimately he just couldn't do it anymore. There's something about being in combat where people's lives are on the line, and then going back to dropping off drug samples in a tissue box that just didn't make him feel like he was contributing, so he left to work for the PGA Tour as a community outreach manager. Shortly after starting his job, Dan decided to have his other leg removed below the knee, which had been long overdue. Following his surgery, Dan spent four more months in recovery and rehab at Walter Reed, and it was the first time in three years Dan felt pain-free.

From there, Dan began to attack life. He climbed Mt. Kilimanjaro, and he began to ride his bike again, traveling all over the country, riding from city to city, putting thousands of miles on it. He eventually left the PGA and started to work for WWP, where he spent seven years. While at WWP, he learned a lot of statistics. For example, 400,000 service members live with PTSD (post-traumatic stress disorder). Dan never really identified with that group because he didn't think he had it, and therefore he never dealt with it. Whenever something came up for Dan as a trigger, he would hop on his bike, pick up his golf clubs, or go for a run or a hike, pushing those thoughts away. He essentially self-medicated through achievement and conquering things. Whether it was leading his team at work or throwing himself into his work, he continued to push those thoughts down deep. Eventually, though, that was no longer a long-term solution.

Dan also learned the statistic that 320,000 service members live with TBI (traumatic brain injury), a group with which he identified due to his own injuries. He also learned that another 53,000 service members were physically wounded in the global war on terror, another statistic with which he identified because his legs were gone. But there was one statistic that he never understood—twenty-two veterans take their own life every single day due to depression and mental illness. Dan had never entertained such an idea himself, not even for a millisecond—that is, until Dan suffered a setback when a recurrent bone infection in his right leg necessitated the amputation of his leg *above* the knee.

Dan had surgery number thirty-six and without batting an eyelash thought, *no big deal, I've done this a million times and recovered from surgery.* The difference this time was that Dan had a job and had to rely on the FMLA (Family Medical Leave Act) to be able to have the surgery and recover. Now divorced, with a three-year-old daughter at home and a job, he decided to fly home to Florida to recover, as opposed to staying at Walter Reed, as he had done in the past. Dan was home alone. He couldn't wear his leg, so he couldn't ride a bike, climb a mountain, or swing a golf club. Hobbling around on two crutches, with one prosthetic leg, Dan couldn't even care for his three-year-old daughter alone anymore. This was the first time Dan felt solitary with his thoughts, and that's when the invisible wounds of war started to surface.

The thoughts Dan used to be able to chase away with a bike ride or with golf clubs came at him every day, omnipresent and intrusive, preventing him from going to sleep. When he would sleep, he would have terrifying nightmares that would wake him up. Finally, Dan realized this was a big problem, and though he never reached the point of being suicidal, for the first time he understood the twenty-two-a-day statistic. Dan realized that he was on his way to becoming one of those twenty-two. He never wanted to live like that and knew he needed help fast. Even though Dan worked for WWP, he was afraid if he called them they would send in the cavalry, breaking down the door to save him. Instead, Dan called his friend Anna for help and recalls her saying what seemed like the stupidest thing he had ever heard anyone say—"You need some yoga in your life." Dan immediately thought *okay, I made a bad decision calling you.*

"I'm a dude. I don't wear spandex. I eat meat and shoot guns. I'm not a hippie, come on now." Unfortunately, that was Dan's perception of yoga. Eventually backing off on the yoga, Anna followed up by saying, "what about meditation?" Dan thought, "Gandhi's cool, what the hell, why not?!" Not knowing what meditation was, Dan spent a while learning from Anna before he started to see real improvements. Not only did the negative thoughts go away, but the quality of the rest of his thoughts improved.

Eight weeks later, he called Anna to thank her for teaching him meditation. Anna followed up by saying "You're welcome, but now you owe me some yoga." "Fine, I'll do your stupid yoga," Dan replied, committing to three private lessons.

Dan's first lesson sucked! It was everything he thought it would be. It was painful, and almost impossible because he was doing it with his prosthetic legs. He made attempts to put his leg out, and bend his knee, but his prosthetic kept jamming in the back of his leg, which brought on sensitivity, since his last surgery was only eight weeks prior. Anna told Dan to "root down, rise up." Not understanding what any of that meant and growing increasingly frustrated, Dan left mad, in pain, and humiliated, not wanting to return. But he had committed to three sessions, and a commitment is a commitment, so Dan went to the second session, and about halfway through he became frustrated again. Dan began having the same issues as the first session, growing frustrated from the pain from his prosthetics. He finally said, "Let me try this with my legs off," which was a big deal because nobody had ever seen Dan without his legs on.

For Dan, before his injury, he felt his best feature was his legs—not his eyes, or his smile, but his legs. Once they were gone, everything changed. People may not understand what happens to an amputee's body after they lose a limb and how everything literally changes in the body. What a person used to consider as the calf muscle on their leg suddenly withers away because there is nothing there. The foot is what now has been replaced to work the leg out, and carry a person's weight. Without having that muscle area there to support the knee, it eventually withers away. To walk, Dan had to use different muscles. He used to have huge quadriceps that would bulge down around his knee caps, but after losing his legs, all the musculature moved up toward his pelvis, so it made his hips wider, still strong, but completely different. They weren't his legs anymore. He would ask himself, "Whose shitty legs are these? These can't be mine."

Dan remembers taking off his legs, getting on his yoga mat, and trying to figure out himself how to proceed. With his knees on his mat, he tried getting into warrior one pose, and he remembered what Anna said, "root down, rise up." And when he consciously thought about being connected, rooting down to the earth, something incredible happened. An energy shot up from the earth into his body as if he were struck by lightning, except there was no pain. It lit Dan up on the inside. He threw his arms in the air, root down, and rose up. Tears started streaming from his eyes, overwhelming him completely because it was actually happening. It wasn't his imagination, it wasn't a story, and he shouted, "Holy shit, this is real." It was as if the earth were saying, "Dan, where have you been for the last ten years?" In that moment, ten years after the blast that changed his life forever, Dan finally let go of the shame in his legs, let go of the need to cover them up.

Even now, after having spent all that time in training, Dan can still feel the connection to the earth with his prosthetics on. Dan says there is nothing that replaces being with his yoga mat and feeling that connection.

Within the last two sessions with Anna, he learned how to adapt to every pose and how to transition, and felt fired up. He committed to doing yoga teacher training, having no intention of being a yoga teacher at all, but simply wanting to learn more. And the more he learned, the more it set him off on his journey, as he wanted to share it with people. Dan's intention was to share the merits of yoga with people like him who think that yoga is either for women, hippies, or weirdos who smell like patchouli oil. Whatever someone's story is of "why *not* to do yoga," he's heard them all and has an answer to all of them why that is simply not true.

There are over 200 styles of yoga, which means that there's a style for everybody. Dan teaches Baptiste Power Vinyasa Yoga, which is great for military folks because it has a militant style but is still 100 percent yoga. Yoga taught Dan so much about himself. Sure, "preyoga" Dan was a nice guy, but even he admits to not being nice all the time. His public face was nice, but he admits that on the inside he didn't always want to be nice and was competitive to a fault.

Now, Dan leads his life with love, trying hard to no longer have prejudgements of people. Each moment and every day is a gift, and each person in Dan's day is a gift. Yoga and meditation also helped Dan realize how amazing his body is, exactly as it is, and exactly as it isn't. Dan now treats his body better, caring about what he puts in it, but admits that he's not perfect. He leads his life the healthiest way he knows how, in his relationships, in what he talks about, and in the decisions he makes that impact other people, not just himself.

What most people don't understand is that being positive is actually a choice. It's a choice we all make, to choose positive even in the most negative situations. Of course it's hard if something negative has happened, or life seems to be against you, but Dan believes you can still choose to be positive. And once you start, it's a snowball effect. Start choosing positive, and you will see the result of your positivity, and the next decision to stay positive is that much easier. The next thing you know, people will ask, "What's different about you?" "What is it?"

For Dan, it's yoga and meditation. But it's not *only* those things; it's a complete shift in the way he sees life. It's about right now. All we have is right now because anything that's already happened, we can't change. It has happened, and there's nothing anyone can do about it. So why spend a single brain cell or a single bit of energy worrying or regretting it? Sure, learn the lesson and take the lesson with you, but not what happened. The worry, fear, doubt, concern, regret, remorse, whatever it is, it won't serve you.

Most people get anxiety over what's going to happen tomorrow, a sense of fear over something that hasn't happened yet. Dan believes that in life there are no guarantees, so why spend the whole day obsessing over it, or stressing over it? It will not serve you. So, if you just live your moment in the now, and make positive choices, right now, then you can create the future you want. Know what you want, and ask yourself the question, "What am I going to do right now?" And then do it. Do one thing! And then tomorrow, do another thing.

The next thing you know, you're eating better, feeling better, you're standing taller, your chest puffs out, your chin is

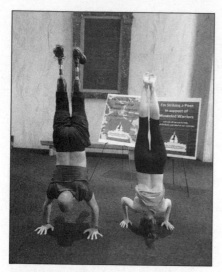

*Dan Nevins and Laurie A. Watkins upside down, U.S. Capitol, Washington, DC.*

up higher, you take better care of yourself, you look five years younger, and you feel ten years younger. People will take notice. Whether it's yoga, Tai Chi, meditation, pushups, or aerobics . . . it's these things that will make all the difference.

## Trauma Can Happen in the Workplace

There were approximately 2.9 million nonfatal workplace injuries and illnesses reported in the U.S. by private industry employers in 2015, which occurred at a rate of 3.0 cases per 100 equivalent full-time workers, according to the U.S. Bureau of Labor Statistics.[36] One industry that has been hit hard over the last few decades is aid workers, and most recently those returning from the frontlines of the Syrian crisis. As a result, the stress and pressures have caused mental health issues. Seventy-nine percent of participants in a Guardian survey of 754 aid staff said they had experienced such conditions, including anxiety, depression, panic attacks, PTSD, and alcoholism.

In 2014, while I was visiting a Syrian refugee camp in Kilis, Turkey, I spoke to "Nancy," Representative, Chief of Mission, at the United Nations High Commissioner for Refugees (UNHCR), who admitted that she had lost about a third of her staff after just one assignment. They quit because of the security risks and emergencies, high workload, extensive travel often in dangerous locations, and separation from their family and friends. All of this came on top of work challenges similar to those faced in other fields, such as an overwhelming number of emails, work/life balance, and difficult colleagues, bosses, and staff.

One way that aid organizations, NGOs, companies, athletic teams, universities, etc., are training their organizations to get unstuck from negative thinking is through the practice of meditation, mindful movement, and ways of understanding and responding to stress. We touched on this earlier in this chapter, but I wanted to provide another example of how meditation can be used to help reduce and relieve work-related stress. This can work for anyone dealing with stress who experiences certain triggers that are making them unhappy and unhealthy, and who may have experienced a trauma in the workplace.

Meditation will give you the tools you need to understand stress and how you can build resilience in the face of the inevitable stresses of life and work, with experiential practices—both formal and informal—that can help build awareness, cultivate greater balance, and strengthen connections with others. These are practices that I engage in myself—and notice when I don't—and I've seen their value for myself and in my work with others. It has also made me a better partner in my personal relationship.

## Stress Release from Laughter? It's No Joke

"Gentlemen, why don't you laugh? With the fearful strain that is upon me day and night, if I did not laugh I should die, and you need this medicine as much as I do." —*Abraham Lincoln, during the Civil War*

With only a few weeks left in the 2012 campaign, and having spent a tremendous amount of time spreading the word about President Obama's space policy along Florida's Space Coast, I knew it would take one last push by a star surrogate to help lock up the vote among college students, who made up a large majority of the vote along the Space Coast. Who better than Bill Nye "The Science Guy"? We had a big job ahead of us. In 2008, Obama barely won those counties that comprise the Space Coast, and with the mandatory retirement of the U.S. Space Shuttle Program in 2010 under the directive of President George W. Bush, our chances seemed slim. Nevertheless, I remained hopeful.

I picked Bill up at the Orlando airport, and from the moment he hopped in my car, we were on one big laugh trip. "You mind if I play some music, Laurie?" he asked, giving me a look from under his sunglasses while taking out his own auxiliary cable from his briefcase. "Not at all," I replied with a smirk, not a bit surprised that the man brought his own gear. Within seconds of his connecting his iPhone to the radio, "Radar Love" by Golden Earring came blaring out of the speakers, causing me to laugh out loud and giving me a high-octane boost that caused me to hit the accelerator full force and send the card speeding along the highway. Bill began dancing from the passenger seat, moving his arms up and down. We were like two kids in high school who had stolen their parents' car for a joyride. And for that brief time, I forgot about the anxiety, stress, and pressure of the job.

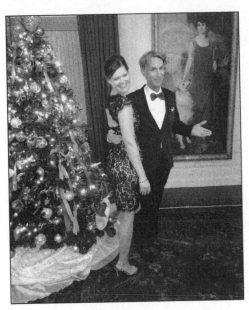

*Bill Nye and Laurie A. Watkins at the White House, Washington, DC.*

Laughing is just one way that Bill relieves stress. Dancing, cycling, surfing, playing ultimate frisbee, and flow activities that involve creating things also make Bill happy. But laughter is essential, and he's made a career out of it by integrating science in an entertaining way that resonates with folks, particularly young people.

After all, laughter isn't just a quick pick-me-up. It's also good for you over the long term. According to the Mayo Clinic, laughter may:

**Improve your immune system.** Negative thoughts, and in turn, stress, decrease your immunity. Positive thoughts, on the other hand, release neuropeptides to fight stress and potentially illness as well.

**Relieve pain.** When you laugh, the body can create its own natural painkillers.

**Increase personal satisfaction.** Plain and simple: laughter connects people.

**Improve your mood.** Laughter has been known to help lessen depression and anxiety.[37]

If you're afraid that your sense of humor is lacking, try these helpful tips offered by the Mayo Clinic:

**Put humor on your horizon.** Find photos, greeting cards, or comic strips—anything that makes you laugh—to hang up at home or in your office. Funny movies, books, comedy albums, joke websites, and visits to a comedy club also help.

**Laugh and the world laughs with you.** Make sure you are laughing. You can even practice, or try laughter yoga. After some practice, it will become more spontaneous.

**Share a laugh.** Spend time with those who make you laugh—and be sure to reciprocate!

**Knock, knock.** Find joke books, and share the humor with those around you.

**Know what isn't funny.** Laughter that hurts someone is not funny. Be able to tell the difference between hurtful humor and good-natured ribbing.[38]

## Trigger Point Release

One of the highest compliments I received after the 2012 presidential campaign came from my colleague and friend Stephanie Young, who went on to become the White House associate communications director, senior public engagement advisor, and primary liaison to the African American community. It was Wednesday, the day after the election, and Stephanie and I were sitting in what had become our favorite nail salon in Tampa, Florida. While sitting with our feet in the basin enjoying a pedicure, Stephanie looked over at me and said, "I really admire how you took time for yourself during this whole thing, putting your foot down when someone tried to take it away. It was impressive, Laurie." To me, that was the highest compliment I could have received because that meant I had won the race—with myself. Before accepting the job as Policy Director for Florida earlier that year, I had had major trepidations about going back to work on a campaign. After all, I had labored over the last few years to lose the campaign weight I gained in 2008, and I had learned to cope with stress through various mechanisms. I vowed to myself right then and there that if I did accept the job, I wouldn't fall into the same, unhealthy habits I had worked so hard to break.

Visits to the nail salon with Stephanie had become a regular thing during the campaign. In a seven-day work week with fourteen-hour days, we had allowed ourselves one hour outside the office, twice a month, to get that one thing done that has become more of a necessity for women (and an increasing number of men) than a luxury (if you happen to work in an industry that judges you based on your appearance), especially in the professional world. Don't get me wrong, the entire hour wasn't all relaxation and bliss. In fact, we frequently walked into the salon already on our phones, earbuds in, balancing a conference call while also furiously answering emails. We always carried our laptops with us, working through the pedicure, but the joy came when we were told to put our devices down, allowing our hands to be free for the manicure and hand massage we so desperately needed.

How a person is groomed can make or break his or her reputation in the business field, especially for women. Stephanie and I were in roles that constantly required us to be up front and personal with very important people, not just sitting in a cubical wearing whatever we threw on that day like most of the staffers at headquarters. Were we supposed to just give up on ourselves and our appearance, chalking it up to "we're on a campaign, who cares?" Hell no! And we knew the VIP folks we were interacting with wouldn't think so either.

A manicured hand is a manicured life, in my opinion. After all, if a man or woman can take care of their nails, they can take care of their work. When a person puts care and attention into something small like their nails, it shows they will put that same care and attention into other aspects of their life. Putting aesthetics aside, manicures are also a great way to take some "me" time. This effort forced us to take a break from our busy lives and relieve the tension and stress of our work.

Lori Garver, former NASA deputy administrator, admits she used to fall flat on how she took care of herself and managed stress. Although she went through most of her career without taking care of herself—putting her kids and job first—she realizes now she should have done a better job. Lori enjoys getting a manicure and a regular massage, taking better care of herself now more than ever before, but admits to being raised by a mother who considered such deeds as decadent, which contributed to her earlier opinions that such activities were unnecessary or perhaps frivolous. Only after seeing and feeling the benefits has she made them a priority. Lori's advice is to do whatever works for you to relieve tension and stress, and to do so in a healthy way.

Christy Adkins, 2016 CrossFit Games competitor, swears by massage to relieve stress. Massage is restorative to the body both physically and mentally, and a large part of how she recovers. Quiet time alone is also incredibly helpful for your mental stress, and Christy recommends finding ways to incorporate that into your schedule.

Whenever someone asks me, "How do you find the time to work out, eat right, or get a massage with your busy schedule?" my response always comes back in the form of a question: "How much time do you take just for yourself each day?" The answers are astounding and mostly the same—either no time at all or somewhere in the range of five to ten minutes. Let's think about that. We all work so incredibly hard at our jobs,

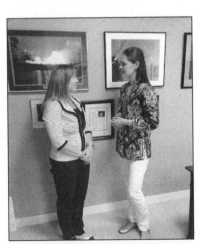

*Lori Garver and Laurie A. Watkins discussing their morning workout routines, Washington, DC.*

taking care of kids, pets, and partners, yet we don't make ourselves a priority. Why not?

Quickly into the 2012 campaign I began feeling the familiar tension and stress in my neck and shoulders, the effects from sitting at my desk for long periods of time, driving long distances across the state of Florida, and enduring the overall pace and long hours of the job. I knew what I had to do. Finding the time to get a massage was not an easy task, but it was a priority to me because it affects my mood and demeanor in a positive way. I wanted to be at my best—not just for me, but for my team.

My CrossFit coach referred me to this amazing masseuse, Emalee, whose studio was only a mile and a half from the office. She was incredibly flexible and understood my hectic schedule, allowing me to book an appointment with little notice. I felt major improvements all around, but the most noticeable was that I was more focused and present with my team. While other colleagues were frequently lashing out at their staff or over the phone with whomever they were speaking to, I remained calm and avoided being easily triggered. I wanted this for the rest of the office.

It wasn't easy, but I found a way to provide twenty blissful minutes to my colleagues by bringing Emalee into campaign headquarters. I pitched the idea to our director that Emalee would be available for half a day, offering twenty-minute time slots of a chair massage to any staffer interested. I told the director that I would handle all of the logistics and everything would be out of sight. No one would ever know that Emalee was there, and it wouldn't disturb anyone's work. Everyone would pay Emalee directly for her services, and there would be no cost to the campaign. It would be a "healthy gesture" that would improve productivity, boost morale, and help manage the stress of the staff. I also told our director that I would sell it to everyone as her idea so she would appear the hero.

I had the go-ahead.

I sent an email to the entire HQ: massage was coming to the office. I gave everyone the details on when Emalee would visit and how to book an appointment. I asked everyone to simply come to my desk and I'd sign them up for a twenty-minute session on my Outlook calendar. Within two minutes of hitting *send*, there was a line around my cube. In fact, the line looked a little crazy at one point, so I asked people to go back to their desks and I would come and find them with their assigned time. All of the available slots were filled in fifteen minutes flat.

Using our office neighbor's conference room downstairs, far away from the noise and crazy ass shenanigans going on upstairs at HQ, Emalee created a makeshift sanctuary. The smell of lavender and sage wafted from the aromatherapy candles she lit on the conference table. Her 2007 portable CD player offered the tranquil sounds of waterfalls and nature. She kept the lighting dim and the mood serene. It was perfect. She had created a "faux spa."

After making sure everyone paid, remained on schedule, and, most important, smiled and felt great as they walked back upstairs to our office—ready to put in another eight hours of work—I went downstairs for my own twenty minutes of silence and relaxation.

My excitement was overwhelming. A guaranteed twenty minutes of uninterrupted silence. It was the only activity I'd had all week when I wasn't required to say a word.

With my face pressed into the paper-covered support of the massage chair, I pretended that my twenty minutes were really sixty. I enjoyed every second of Emalee kneading out knots and kinks, massaging away all the stress, worry, and tension I was holding in my shoulders and neck. I was carrying stress from the campaign, stress from being away from home and my dog, tension in my muscles from CrossFit and running, and most of all I was holding the painstaking stress from trying to survive in this all-consuming life of a presidential campaign.

For those twenty minutes, I let everything go. I closed my eyes and quickly fell asleep. I woke up feeling renewed, fresh, and lighter than before.

Along with the coffee in the office kitchen, chatter was brewing early the next morning. The people who had paid for a chair massage went around the office chatting with colleagues, telling them how much better they felt this morning and how they were going to commit to regularly rewarding their bodies with a massage. My inbox was full from people thanking me for bringing Emalee in, asking me for her contact information. My plan had worked even better than I had envisioned, but I did not want to become Emalee's booker. So I posted her business card on the kitchen bulletin board and said, "Go nuts."

A few hours later, I got an email from Emalee, who had already received half a dozen inquiries from staff members to schedule appointments the following week. With regular appointments, I was confident that my colleagues would see all kinds of benefits—increased circulation of blood and lymph fluids of the body, relief from muscular tension, acute stress relief, enhanced immunity, and regulation of blood pressure. Our bodies work hard for us each and every day of our lives. We expect years of service from them, years that are often filled with too little sleep, too little exercise, bad food, bad air, bad water, and so much stress. Yet how often do we pay attention to the signals of wear and tear that our bodies send through an aching back, sore shoulders, and a stiff neck?

Massage therapy is great because it helps you to reconnect with your body. That's what I was hoping for my colleagues when I came up with the idea. My thinking was that if I brought in a professional who could help show them how to relieve stress and tension, there would be no opportunity for excuses like they didn't have time, couldn't leave the office, or had too much to do. Their overall health and well-being would be improved while their stress levels decreased. They would become more productive, happier people. And that's the kind of people I wanted to work with!

## Reduce Your Stress in the Great Outdoors

My favorite way to chill out, relax, and get recentered is by being outdoors, in nature and all of its glorious splendor. Perhaps it's because my parents took my brother and me to State and National Parks for as far back as I can remember, choosing nature versus the barrage of expensive and crowded theme parks that were located only a few hours away from where I grew up in Florida. As an adult I came to appreciate the gift they gave us, looking forward to opportunities of exploring the world's natural landscape and our National Parks, on my own terms.

Jake Frank, ranger, National Park Service, will never forget the first time he drove into the Tetons, moving into his new house with the Grand Canyon located directly behind it, thinking, "This is unbelievable!"[39] Whether it was when he first arrived at Glacier National Park among mountains strewn as far as the eye could see, the first time he laid eyes on the Grand Canyon, or his first time going down into the Hawaii Volcanoes at night as the earth glowed bright into the sky with the Milky Way above it, these are memories and feelings simply too awesome to describe. Jake admits that he's never gotten a feeling like that from any other source; the awe of nature and its grandeur make him feel small, but also put things into perspective.

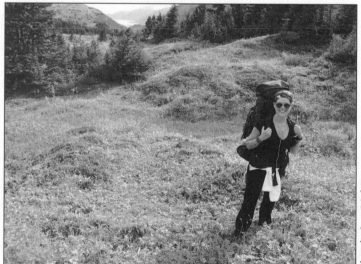

Photo by Scott Watkins

*Laurie A. Watkins backpacking along Lost Lake Trail, Kenai Peninsula, Alaska.*

We're all animals, having evolved from the natural world, and when in nature, we use all of our senses to survive. When we are inside, we don't hear bird sounds or feel the grass under our feet. By going into the parks, Jake says we have the opportunity to do those things—hear the natural sounds of running water, wind, and birds, and the rustle of trees and branches. Jake cautions that when you first go out there, you may not know what you're hearing because you have been deprived of it for so long. The longer you stay, you can start to really hear the birds, and if you sit and close your eyes, you will start to hear and feel the many layers of things happening around you that a lot of the time we simply aren't tuned into.

David Strayer, cognitive psychologist at the University of Utah who specializes in attention, knows our brains are prone to mistakes, especially when we're multitasking and dodging distractions. Our brains, he says, aren't tireless three-pound machines; they're easily fatigued. When we slow down, stop the busywork, and take in beautiful natural surroundings, not only do we feel restored, but our mental performance improves too. Strayer is in a unique position to understand what modern life does to us. An avid backpacker, he thinks he knows the antidote: Nature. "If you can have the experience of being in the moment for two or three days, it seems to produce a difference in qualitative thinking," he explained in an interview with *National Geographic*. Strayer's hypothesis is that being in nature allows the prefrontal cortex, the brain's command center, to dial down and rest, like an overused muscle. "At the end of the day," he says, "we come out in nature not because the science says it does something to us, but because of how it makes us feel."[40]

When the stress from work plagues Jake, he says there's nothing like going outside on a hike, watching the sun rise or set, or going for a walk and just listening to what's around him to eliminate his stress. Being outside doesn't necessarily require you to be active, but Jake says if you keep moving, it can help lower your stress levels more so than simply sitting still. Nothing will put you in a better mood than taking in something beautiful. Try hanging out at a lake, swimming, going on a hike, or even summiting a peak; these are all recommendations to help improve your mood, making you happier and more pleasant to be around.

I realize for some, visiting one of our National Parks may bring a lot of questions, even fears: "The parks seem so far away, I don't have anyone to go with, it's too expensive, I've never been camping, will I be safe, what if I don't own any gear?" The NPS (National Park Service) understands and has worked extremely hard over the years to help eliminate and answer these questions. Through the 2016 Centennial and Find Your Park initiative, they aim to bring awareness that there are over four hundred National Parks located all over the country, with at least one National Park in each state, whether it's a battlefield or a seashore. Most of the parks can be visited in one day, or even in a few hours.

The NPS has figured out ways of connecting with a new and younger generation of visitors and potential visitors through social media, reaching beyond the traditional demographics of baby boomers, retirees, nonminorities, and folks already familiar with the parks. It has hosted

InstaMeets via Instagram, where anyone can come and meet other people, hang out, and have a shared experience with those who happen to be in the same place at the same time, or do their own research online by looking at photos and deciding, "Wow, that's really cool, I want to go there." These are all examples of how you can easily get outside, and have a great time, most of the time for free. When people share their amazing photos and stories with friends through social media, they are helping to carry on the intention and tradition of why the NPS was even created one hundred years ago—to promote the fact that these places are real, and we need to protect them. The majority of people in the U.S. back then weren't able to see these awesome places because they were so far away in the West or hadn't yet been explored, and in order to show members of Congress back in DC that these places did in fact exist and needed to be preserved, artists and photographers were sent there in order to bring stories back to share.

There's a reason why people keep going back to visit our National Parks (some even choose to get engaged and married inside). Whether it's for the emersion into deep, rich history, views of the beautiful vistas, or the peaceful feeling one gets while being there, they just make you feel good. Throughout Jake's career, he's met people from all walks of life who have shared their stories and experiences regarding what brought them to the park. Whether it was being able to capture a friend's engagement in Rocky Mountain National Park, eventually marrying them in Alaska; listening to the story of a former ultra-runner, now paralyzed, who used a handcycle to hike through Glacier

National Park; or happening to stumble upon Daniel as he crossed the 16,000-mile mark, walking across the United States. We all have a story, but the common thread is that it doesn't matter where you're from, how old you are, your gender, sexuality, or race; being in nature feeds the spirit, affects our brains and bodies in a positive way, and makes us happy and less stressed.

# CHAPTER 6

# PROTECT YOUR WORKOUT BY MAKING IT A PRIORITY

Hopefully throughout the course of this book, you have learned that the mind and body are in fact interrelated. Your mental state affects your ability to physically function, just as your level of physical fitness affects your emotional well-being.

By now, we should all know that maintaining an active lifestyle should be a top priority. Only when we take care of ourselves do we have hope for success in being the kind of person we strive to be at home, at work, and in our communities.

Our jobs can definitely get in the way of working out—but only if we let them. Sure, we all struggle to find time to exercise, but the reality is that we can't afford not to work out. The "high achievers" and high-powered folks who have shared their stories throughout the book somehow managed to live a healthy, well-balanced life, no matter what challenges were thrown at them. What will it take for you to do the same?

To make getting started easier, I have put together some tips for how to fit working out into your daily routine, no matter how demanding your job may be. No one should settle for less than feeling healthy, strong, and capable of doing whatever their heart desires. I'll be honest with you: this will not happen overnight. But, I do promise that you'll feel a difference almost immediately.

### 1. Work Out Efficiently

Pick a type of workout that you can do from almost anywhere, whether you're traveling or getting home late from the office. This should be a form of exercise that doesn't require much planning or equipment. Since your time is valuable, you can't waste one second on a bad workout—the good ones are tough enough to plan for. Running, bodyweight exercises, Tabata training, and yoga are all stellar choices. In terms of preparation, there are things you can do to improve your efficiency and strength during the workouts—make sure you are well rested, you have enough energy, your playlist is ready to go, and you always have enough water to drink before, during, and after.

Bill Nye has been faithful to his workout regimen five to six days a week for the last four years. "You've gotta make time for it, that's the hardest challenge," he says. Bill, who lives in New York City, finds working out around 5:30 or 6 o'clock in the evening in his building's gym to be the best time, since no one is around, with many New Yorkers still at work.

Besides spending time in the gym, Bill enjoys cycling (you may even catch him riding around NYC on one of the Citi Bikes) and dancing. Long before his days on "Dancing with the Stars," Bill participated in ballroom and swing dancing regularly from 1978 to 1998 while living in Seattle. He never considered it to be exercise, but rather a bonus because of how much fun it was. Whether it's at a conventional venue in Pasadena, New York, London, Tokyo, or San Francisco, Bill says dancing is extremely athletic, and you can expect to dance for almost three hours, leaving with a soaked, sweaty shirt. "The music gets fast, what are you gonna do?!" he says.

Bill's favorite part of dancing . . . holding the woman. "It's fantastic," he says with a grin. Sometimes you get a partner that sees it the way you do. Dancing is a conversation; there's the beat, and then there's either side of the beat, and we're talking about fractions of seconds. The best is when you find a partner that can get on that same fraction of a second, as if you're both watching the same invisible conductor.

A few months before going on season seventeen of "Dancing with the Stars," Bill began working out, particularly his upper body. Unfortunately, only three weeks into the competition, Bill suffered a serious leg injury, tearing his quadriceps tendon during a taped rehearsal. Going against his doctor's advice, Bill danced anyway to the creative jazz choreography created by partner Tyne Stecklein, which allowed him to wear a leg immobilizer, sticking mostly to hand movements. In the end, Bill was eliminated and extremely disappointed.

During a visit by the show's sports medicine doctor following the incident, Bill was told that his age had contributed to the injury. Motivated to recover without surgery, Bill began a disciplined regimen of physical therapy and exercise, eventually becoming stronger than before the injury. Concerned about his posture after years of abuse to his spine that began when he was a young man (hunched down, not wanting to appear taller than his classmates) and was aggravated during many years of long-distance cycling, Bill decided to supercharge his workout routine, lifting heavier weights, and eventually grew increasingly stronger in his core and back.

Bill starts his workout by warming up on a bike for ten minutes. He then stretches for ten minutes and then does some crunches while holding either a bar or a medicine ball. He rounds out the workout with what he calls the "Rafalski Shuffle," which is a take on the abdominal scissor kick that he named after his trainer, Jesse Rafalski. It is crucial to stretch before performing any physical activity to prevent injury, increase range of motion, and increase blood flow to the muscles.

## Rafalski Shuffle

### Step 1: Starting Position

Lie on your back on an exercise mat with your legs side by side and extended. Place your fingertips on your head just behind your ears to provide a little support for your head. Lift your head and shoulder blades off the mat. Hover your heels a couple of inches off the mat.

### Step 2: Contract Your Core Muscles

Press your lower back firmly into the mat and slightly tuck your pelvis. Draw your belly button in toward your spine. Maintain this position throughout the exercise.

### Step 3: Initiate the Movement

Move your legs in a vertical plane to create the scissoring action. As your right leg lifts up, your left leg lowers to hover above the mat. Keep your legs as straight as possible.

**Step 4: Add the Twist**

As your right leg rises, rotate your torso to the right, bringing your left elbow toward your right thigh. Your left shoulder blade will come higher off the ground, and your right shoulder blade may touch the mat. Return to center as your legs pass each other, then rotate your torso to the left as your left leg rises.

Bill then does a WOD (workout of the day) while jamming out to a playlist. Some of his favorite songs include: "Days Go By" (Dirty Vegas), "Mystery Train" (Elvis Presley), "Double Shot of My Baby's Love" (Swingin' Medallions), and "You Shook Me" (Led Zeppelin). To help get you started, Bill shares a **three- and four-day workout**, designed especially for you, with help from his trainer, Jesse. "Go change the world," Bill instructs.

## 3-DAY SEQUENCE

*Each day, perform 3 sets of each group before moving on to the next group

Total of 27 sets each day, 3 sets per activity (9 sets per group)

## DAY ONE:

(10-minute bike warm-up)

Stretch

Group 1:

PUSH-UPS, 25 Flat or Inclined

INCLINED FLIES, 20 reps

STANDING CHEST FLIES, 20 reps

Group 2:

CRUNCHES (bench with heavy ball overhead), 50

MILITARY PRESS, 20 reps
SEATED SIDE RAISES, 20 reps
Group 3:
STANDING CURLS, 20 reps
BENCH DIPS, 30 reps
SEATED HAMMER CURLS, 20 reps

## DAY TWO:
(10-minute bike warm-up)
Stretch
Group 1:
SEATED WIDE GRIP PULLDOWNS, 20 reps
SEATED ROWS, 20 reps
CLOSE-GRIP PULLDOWNS, 20 reps
Group 2:
SHRUGS, 20 reps with barbell
DEADLIFTS, 20 reps with barbell
ROPE-TO-THE-THROAT STANDING PULLS, 20 reps
Group 3:
CRUNCHES, 50
REVERSE BENCH FLYES, 20 reps
STANDING FRONT RAISES, 20 reps

## DAY THREE:
(10-minute bike warm-up)
Stretch
Group 1:
LEG EXTENSIONS, 25 reps
SQUATS, 25
RAFALSKI SHUFFLE, 50

Group 2:
PUSH-UPS, 25
INCLINED DUMBBELL PRESS, 20 reps
INCLINED FLYES, 20 reps
Group 3:
CLOSE GRIP TRICEP PUSH-UPS, 20 reps
PREACHER CURLS, 20 reps
FRONT RAISES, STRAIGHT ARM, 20 reps each side

# 4-DAY REGIMEN FOR BUILDING MUSCLE MASS

### Isolated Muscle Groups

*Pick weights where you can start with 12 reps (going down in reps if necessary)

## DAY ONE (Chest):

(10-minute warm-up on the bike)
Stretch
DUMBBELL PRESS, 4 sets, increasing weight each set
INCLINED PRESS, 4 sets, increasing weight each set
PUSH-UPS, 4 sets of 20
CRUNCHES, BENCH & HEAVY BALL (held overhead), 50
STANDING CHEST FLYES, 4 sets

## DAY TWO (Back):

(10-minute warm-up on the bike)
Stretch
WIDE-GRIP PULL-DOWNS, 4 sets, increasing weight each set

CLOSE GRIP PULL-DOWNS, 4 sets, increasing weight each set
ROW, 4 sets, increasing weight each set
CRUNCHES, RAFALSKI SHUFFLE, 50
PULL-UPS (as many as possible until failure)

## DAY THREE (Shoulders):
(10-minute warm-up on the bike)
Stretch
MILITARY PRESS, 4 sets, increasing weight each set
SEATED SIDE RAISES, 4 sets, increasing weight each set
REVERSE FLYES, INCLINED BENCH, 4 sets, increasing weight each set
FRONT RAISES, 4 sets, increasing weight each set
CRUNCHES, BENCH & HEAVY STRAIGHT BAR (held overhead), 50

## DAY FOUR (Arms):
(10-minute warm-up on the bike)
Stretch
STANDING CURLS, 4 sets, increasing weight each set
ROPE PUSH-DOWNS, 4 sets, increasing weight each set
CLOSE GRIP PUSH-UPS, 4 sets of 25
BENCH DIPS, 4 sets of 30
HAMMER CURLS, 4 sets, increasing weight each set
CRUNCHES, FLAT MAT, 50

### 2. Sign Up for Competitions as Motivation
Starting something new can be a big challenge for most people, and sticking with it can be an even bigger challenge.

When we're trying to motivate ourselves to exercise regularly, competition can be just the thing to light a fire under us. Nothing can kick-start your focus and training more than signing up for a competition. The desire to "get fit by X date" should certainly get you moving, and by signing up for an obstacle course, CrossFit competition, 5K, or half marathon, you have something to motivate you as you work toward your goal, whether it's simply finishing or placing in your age group. No one will know more than you if you don't put in the training time.

Phil Larson holds himself accountable this way by signing up for half marathons, keeping his focus on race day, and putting in the miles necessary for a successful race. It's as simple as adding a work reminder to your calendar on training days and logging the miles you did that day in the notes section. By tracking your activity and time, you can monitor your progress and see where, if any, there is still room for improvement. For Phil, while he was at the White House, he focused mainly on diet and losing the weight, while doing moderate exercise, which helped eliminate pounds as well as pain. He was then able to run on all cylinders, focusing more on high-intensity interval training and running. "You have to just decide to do it, no matter how hard it may be to carry out," he explains. After you start, you'll realize that it really didn't take that much time out of your day. Try refocusing your priorities, and eliminate things that don't serve you.

Being self-motivated is hard—so how about sweating for donations to your favorite charity with either colleagues or friends? You become accountable to the people who give you money, the people who are cheering you on, your colleagues and team members, and most important, the people and organization you are trying to help. Try signing up for a charity run or enlisting to run a marathon on behalf of a cause. I promise you will have fun while doing it!

### 3. Make a Schedule and Commit to It

After the 2008 presidential campaign in Florida, I found myself working in the Pentagon. Books primed me for the difference between military and civilian culture, the length of time it took actions to go up the long chain of command, and how to effectively navigate the surprisingly confusing building. What the books didn't prepare me for was the culture of fitness. Working out, even during the middle of the workday, wasn't just allowed—it was encouraged. These workouts weren't mild-mannered jogs either.

The motivation, encouragement, and inspiration by people running the building changed my way of thinking for the rest of my life. That way of thinking was put to the test early on during the 2012 campaign when our Press Secretary threatened to fire me if I left the office to work out. Respectfully, I called his bluff and went anyway. You can keep putting everything and everyone else before you, or you can choose yourself. The former means a life likely full of illness, injuries, and pains. The latter steers you toward a life of happiness, adventure, and independence into old age. The obvious answer is to start making exercise your #1 priority *right now.*

I didn't fold under pressure as most probably would have, thanking the heavens above that their boss just eighty-sixed their evening workout. Instead, I guarded that time like a mother tiger guards her cubs and said, "No, I can do that when I get back from the gym." Guarding my own time—and sometimes being a little selfish—was the key to keeping my stress in check during that long, busy stretch of the campaign. It made me a better person, coworker, and friend—and it can work for others, too.

But no matter how hard you try, no one can force you to take that path. You have to want it badly enough. You have to choose it for yourself.

You can feed your body junk and make all the excuses you can think of to avoid exercising, or you can start eating right and working out regularly and with purpose.

### 4. Satisfy Your Own Likes and Dislikes

Make it easier on yourself by choosing a form of exercise that not only fits your schedule, but also your lifestyle and personality. Do you prefer working out on your own or being part of a group exercise class? If you work out on your own, you can set your own schedule, pace, and workout location. But if you're someone like me who needs motivation and enjoys working out with people and having a coach that helps keep you accountable, then I recommend joining a gym class. Whether you choose spinning, yoga, CrossFit, Pilates, or dance, don't be afraid to experiment until you find what works for you. Maybe you're a person who likes more than one form of exercise. By diversifying your routine, you work different muscle groups and areas of the body, leading to a healthier, happier you.

I realize that some people may feel self-conscious, so I recommend choosing a beginner class or starting at home with a convenient online streaming option until you feel more confident. There are tons of resources on the Web that offer free classes and low-cost monthly subscriptions guaranteed to get you good and sweaty.

After the 2012 presidential campaign was over and I moved back to Washington, I was invited to become a member of the exclusive RunBrunch group. Its exclusivity was built on the fact that two Chicago Obama alumni, Dan and Alexis, created a home (posse) of Obama alumni who liked to run and brunch. Every week an email would go out to the group with a route for the run (5-7 miles for the "rabbits" and 1-3 miles for the "beach cruisers") and a location for brunch afterwards. Eventually, what started out as a once-a-week meet-up turned into a solid group of friends and colleagues who hung out more than just on "run day." We ran half-marathons and 5Ks together, had printed t-shirts and sunglasses made, and held annual Christmas parties. It was great and a fantastic way to exercise with friends and have fun while doing it.

Between her two tours at NASA, Lori Garver, who worked as an independent consultant (which provided a flexible schedule and more time to spend with her kids), had her own fitness regimen. Every Saturday morning, Lori attended an aerobics class that included a large group of stay-at-home and work-from-home moms from the neighborhood who always went out for coffee together afterwards. These women were really good at knowing when sign-ups were for soccer, swim lessons, piano, how to get on the wait list at the community pool, who the best teachers were to request at school, etc., and became Lori's lifeline, where she got all of her information.

One Saturday, the aerobics instructor announced she was leaving the area and unless someone stepped up to teach the class, it would be cancelled. The other moms didn't care if the group died a premature death or not, but Lori certainly cared. How would she stay informed or get in that workout with the ladies she looked forward to seeing every week? She panicked when her attempt to get one of the moms to become certified and teach the class failed. There was only one other option—Lori would have to do it herself.

Even as the only full-time working mom in the group, she couldn't afford to lose the opportunity of gathering with these women once a week, so Lori went and got certified to teach aerobics. She had to study anatomy charts and human kinetics and spent three days in Atlantic City to obtain her certification. She ended up teaching the class for six years and was able to keep the coffee clutch going, retaining contacts with her kids' friends' mothers even after they went off to college. Lori says it wasn't easy, but she did what she had to do, adjusting her schedule and priorities for something she enjoyed.

### 5. Start with ONE thing. It's Better to Choose Something over Nothing

Take a few minutes to think about what it is that you would like to change about yourself, making it easier to reach your goal of improving your health and identity. Do you want to be able to cook healthy meals during the workweek? Do you want to be able to work out in the morning before heading to the office? Do you want to lose that stubborn weight around your mid-section? What's stopping you?

Once you've determined what you want, it's time to start working on it with small, realistic wins, proving to yourself that you can change and are capable of making healthier, more impactful choices. By picking ONE part of that new identity, and focusing all of your effort and willpower on proving to yourself that in fact you are capable of turning it into a reality, you will gain the motivation you need to make even more changes, building better habits.

I do not recommend making drastic, unrealistic declarations to yourself like "I'm going to work out seven days a week and lose thirty pounds in a month." This will only crush you when it doesn't happen, causing you to lose the motivation to continue the hard work you've already put in.

If you have a goal of being able to get up early enough in the morning to work out, but hit the snooze button every time, then start out by going to bed one hour earlier each night for a week, even before you try going to the gym. If you drink soda and want to quit, but find it hard because of the sugar and caffeine addiction, try drinking one fewer can each day during that week, eventually eliminating the soft drink completely from your diet. My recommendation is to pick one thing and fix it before moving on to the next. Make it something you can measure, something that you're able to check off your list, realizing, "Wow, I accomplished X this week."

To get a complete workout, you don't need an hour, or even thirty minutes, for it to be effective. Some exercise is better than nothing, so if you need to start small, that's okay. If you establish an effective program, done consistently, both short and long workouts can do wonders for your body, mind, and spirit. These small gains at the start will help prove to yourself that you can make a lifelong change by creating a new pattern, a new normal.

After Jamie Leeds started losing all the weight she had carried for years, she was overwhelmed by the energy she had, which was sometimes so intense that her body only allowed her to stay asleep for three to four hours at a time. She had to start small, easing her way into running and cycling again. It didn't happen overnight, but she was patient, listening to her body, focusing on small gains and building from there.

For those who keep putting themselves off, neglecting your health and well-being with the excuse that you just don't have time, energy, resources, etc., accept that you can't do it alone. You need support, whether that comes from a friend, partner, trainer, or even a coworker. If you want to start an exercise routine, but don't know how, Jamie recommends getting a trainer or someone other than yourself who is going to get you into the gym and hold you accountable. Even though you made the appointment, and may have already paid for the session, you have to show up. That is where the hard work comes in. You can't let the other person do the work for you. And if you already work out in a gym or fitness center, but don't feel you're seeing results, consider asking the on-site personal trainer to work with you for a few weeks, establishing a training plan to teach you proper form and technique.

I would love to say that you can do it alone, but it's simply not true. You need to create a support system around you. Whether it's asking your spouse or partner to get the kids up in the morning while you go to the gym, or hiring a trainer in the beginning to help design a plan aligned with your goals and that works for your body and capabilities, it's impossible to do it alone. And if you don't have the resources to hire a trainer, ask a friend for assistance. Try running with a neighbor or coworker before or after work. Just don't be afraid to ask for help. All it takes is ONE change in habit to create the positive difference to remain motivated for success.

### 6. If You Don't Measure It, It Doesn't Exist

Measuring your activity levels and keeping notes on your progress can help you stay on track and realize when you're stumbling before the habit is completely gone. Paying attention to how your body is responding to your fitness program can also help you make changes and tweaks along the way. Whether your goal is to lose weight or gain muscle, you'll find it easier to stay on course with some type of tracking system in place. Here are some recommendations to make tracking your progress easier:

1.  Take before and after pictures with the same pose and outfit, making sure to time stamp each photo.
2.  Keep a journal and write down the workout and result. If you lift weights, this will help you remember the appropriate weight for next time, while also keeping track of your last PR (personal record). If you run, log your miles and time. I also recommend recording your mood that day, as it can impact your workout and explain any fluctuation.

3. Weigh yourself. I don't recommend doing this very often because you risk the chance of driving yourself crazy. Only do this at certain milestones, e.g., 30, 60, 90 days, to track progress.

4. Pay attention to how your clothes fit. If they start feeling loose, you're on the right track.

5. Take circumference measurements (again, at different milestones) to track your waist, hips, and abdominal girth. This is helpful, for example, if your weight hasn't changed but you've dropped one or two pant sizes. This will demonstrate that you've gained muscle and lost fat.

6. Use a mobile app. These are ideal assistants for health, fitness, and weight loss because they're always with us, and quite personal. Fitness trackers such as Moov Now, AppleWatch, FitBit, Jawbone, Misfit, or Garmin are also helpful options but require you to wear them 24/7. There's definitely something out there for everyone.

"By tracking your individual progress, you afford yourself the opportunity to make progress," says West Point cadet Austin Willard. Running a lot is a requirement in the military, and to keep himself on point, Willard writes down how far he went, how fast he ran, and where. He uses this data to help improve his performance for the next run. If you like to lift weights and you're benching the barbell, write down what you benched the bar at, and how many reps you got, then try and do more the next time.

It's especially important for people who are just getting started that they not get discouraged when they see someone who's been doing something for years and compare themselves. That's not being fair to yourself, so don't do it. Maintain realistic expectations, and track your progress, making sure you steadily improve. Don't expect after only two months that you're going to the CrossFit Games and winning "Fittest person on earth." Keep a long-term perspective, understanding that it's going to take months and years to make significant and noticeable progress. If you accept that results will not happen overnight, and continue to take care of yourself physically, the hard work will pay dividends. If you don't take care of yourself, you won't be useful to anyone, especially yourself.

### 7. Don't Be Afraid to Ask for Help

There are many possible reasons that might be influencing your reluctance to seek help from others. One is your concern about how others view you, or that you don't want to inconvenience someone. Do you battle with fears of rejection or have a tendency toward perfectionism? All of these motivations can cause you to avoid accepting help, for fear of failing or being seen as a failure. If you're a professional or business owner, you may be worried that needing help can demonstrate a lack of professionalism or even be seen as a sign of weakness. Consequently, you might feel that someone not handling their own affairs is inferior or incompetent. The same goes for managing your exercise schedule, health, and wellness.

For Christy Adkins, 2016 CrossFit Games competitor, even though she has the drive to compete and be the best in her sport, she gives herself credit that she has the ability to reach out to others, asking for help. Just like me and you, she doesn't always feel mentally strong, and asking for help can come in the form of coaches with various specialties, such as gymnastics, Olympic weightlifting for fuller body workouts, swimming, chiropractic care, and more. These folks all provide a greater depth of experience, more than simply teaching a skill. They've also helped Christy with mental gains.

In 2015, Christy suffered the biggest loss of her career by not qualifying for the CrossFit Games. With the loss affecting her mental state and confidence, she hired a mental game coach, as she trained for the 2016 Games. For Christy, it was important to be able to admit to those closest to her how she was really feeling. Being able to talk to her husband, sister, and parents and admitting total vulnerability was where she found the strength to be able to speak about her fears and doubts with other people.

If you are struggling with personal issues like time management or finding motivation to work out, asking for help is not limited to just your immediate close circle of friends, but a larger support network. Talk to other professionals; they've probably been through the same problems and would be happy to help you. They have a wealth of knowledge, and it's quite possible that their experience might give you the extra dose of perspective that you need to start making progress. The point here is not to limit yourself in whom you can ask for help. Take a hard look at what resources are available to you and who can help you accomplish your goals and make the very most of them.

Don't let pride or fear get in the way of gleaning everything you can from your workout experience. Taking the time to identify what you need and how to get it is never a waste of time. This is your life, and it's up to you to get the most from this experience.

# CHAPTER 7

# TIME MANAGEMENT

**tomorrow**

(*noun*)

A MYSTICAL LAND WHERE 99% OF ALL HUMAN
PRODUCTIVITY, MOTIVATION, AND ACHIEVEMENT IS STORED

-AUTHOR UNKNOWN

I don't have time. I'll get to it later. Time is money. I wish there were more hours in the day. I'll be there in five minutes. I always feel like I'm rushing to get somewhere.

Do any of these phrases sound familiar? Well, they should, because most of us experience stress and that uneasy feeling as if we have a perceived lack of control over the daily events in our lives. Time management means exactly that— managing one's time. But, don't worry, you're not alone.

In 2013, McKinsey and Company asked nearly 1,500 executives across the globe to tell them how they spent their time; they found that only 9 percent of the respondents deemed themselves "very satisfied" with their current allocation. Less than half were "somewhat satisfied," and about one-third were "actively dissatisfied." What's more, only 52 percent said that the way they spent their time largely matched their organizations' strategic priorities. Nearly half admitted that they were not concentrating sufficiently on guiding the strategic direction of the business.[41]

The survey results, while disquieting, are arguably a natural consequence of the fact that few organizations treat executive time as the finite and measurable resource it is. Leadership time, by contrast, too often gets treated as though it were limitless, with all good opportunities receiving high priority regardless of the leadership capacity to drive them forward. No wonder so few leaders feel they are using their time well.

The biggest and most destructive myth regarding time management is that you can get everything done if only you follow the right system, use the right to-do list, or process your tasks in the right way. That's a mistake. As the 19th-century thinker Henry David Thoreau wrote, "It is not enough to be busy. So are the ants."

If you want to take back control of your workday schedules and priorities, the only way to do it is by relentlessly questioning how you're spending your time. I always like to start with this question: What are you doing in this moment?

The simple act of becoming more aware of where your attention is going will help you focus it where you want it to be—on achieving your compelling goals. Too often we get distracted or get caught up in unimportant tasks that end up wrecking our day and derailing our to-do lists. The ways you feel about the tasks you hate doing are big, red flags that encourage you to find a way to pass those unpleasantries on to someone or something (like a system) that can tackle them for you. But first, you've gotta figure out exactly what's making you crazy in the first place.[42]

The first honest question you must ask yourself is "How am I using my time?" We must be cognizant of how we portion our time, use our time effectively, and with whom we choose to spend that precious time. Only then will we feel a sense of control. Strength is not just physical; it is mental, too. By following these time management recommendations, you'll be on your way to feeling stronger, more in control, and less uneasy throughout your day.

## Smart Time Management Tools

1. Do the most important thing first every day. It sounds simple, but most of us don't do it. For me, I choose working out to start my day because it makes me feel energized, motivated, and accomplished even if it's before seven o'clock in the morning.

2. Make a list, and actually use it. Set reminders on your phone or computer, and if they happen more than once a week/month, set them as recurring events, making sure you're covered. Before going to bed at night, review your calendar for the following day to avoid scrambling the next morning.

3. Favor trusting relationships. Put effort into building relationships with people you can trust and count on, and make sure those same people can trust and count on you. If there's someone in your life who constantly cancels after making plans, get rid of them. It may sound harsh, but ask yourself, would you allow your significant other, spouse, or partner to get away with

that type of disrespect? The answer is "no." So why let a friend or colleague do the same?

4. Be on time. If you're always running five to fifteen minutes late in an eight-hour work day, that's potentially two hours wasted. Subtract that from the total time you initially planned to complete the long to-do list created earlier that morning, and you'll find yourself in big trouble.

5. Be authentic. Be as honest with yourself as you can about what you want and why you do what you do. Don't remain involved with organizations, groups, or boards that don't fulfill your passion but instead suck the life out of you, wasting your time.

6. Get good at saying no to other people, and do so frequently. Turn down things that are inconsistent with your priorities. This has been the hardest for me to stick to because I tend to feel bad when I have to decline an invitation, but it's forced me to ask myself, "Does this fall in line with your priorities or goals?" If the answer is no, then your response to the invitation should be the same, "No."

7. Maintain a lifestyle that will give you maximum energy. Work your way up to exercising at least three times a week, eating a healthy lunch, drinking plenty of water, and getting enough sleep. If you need to be at work early in the morning and remain sharp throughout the day, going out all night is probably not the best choice.

8. Listen to your biorhythms (as Dr. Kotler recommended earlier in the book) and organize your day

accordingly. Make it a habit to pay attention to regular fluctuations in your physical and mental energy levels throughout the day; based on how you feel, make adjustments to how you schedule tasks.

9.  Set very few priorities and stick to them. Select a maximum of two things that are your highest priority and plan time to work on them. No one wants a twenty-five-item to-do list, where at the end of the day you look at it realizing you've only checked off four or five items.

10. Set specific time slots to answer email. If you stick to this, you won't be distracted when yet another email pops up in your inbox, fighting for your attention and energy. If you have the type of job where you have to answer or acknowledge email right away, spend no more than five minutes and move on.

11. Stop overscheduling yourself. Having a jam-packed schedule five days a week doesn't allow for the unexpected occurrence like a dinner or coffee with a friend who comes to town, scheduling that dentist appointment or haircut, picking up the dry cleaning, or getting that massage you so desperately need, but for which you simply don't have a time slot.

12. Always look for ways of doing things better and faster. Be on the lookout for tasks you do over and over again and look for ways of improving how you do them. Don't be afraid to ask for help. Delegation is not a sign of weakness, but a sign of intelligence. Find competent, reliable people and share some of the

responsibilities. It will allow you to be less stressed and more productive.

13. Build solid processes. Set up processes that last and run without your attention—whether that means letting go and delegating tasks to a colleague or trusting that the procedure you set up will operate efficiently without you. Avoid the need to "check in" so much.

14. Finish what's important and stop doing what's no longer worthwhile. Don't stop doing what you considered worth starting unless there's a good reason to throw in the towel. When you realize that one of your goals is going to require extra effort, eliminate that which doesn't serve the mission.

15. Reward yourself. When you finish a task or complete a project, celebrate your accomplishments. Of course it's best to do things in moderation and in a healthy way, but treating yourself to a nice meal, a night out with friends, or an epic vacation are things that will help motivate you the next time you come up against a challenging task.

## Create Your Own Space within Your Organization

Lori Garver began working for the National Space Institute after her boss, John Glenn, got out of the presidential race. During her fourteen-year tenure there as Executive Director, she earned a master's degree at night in International Science and Technology Policy from George Washington University.

Along with the pressures of being the Executive Director came the responsibility of regularly testifying in front of Congress. At the age of twenty-seven, she also had two small boys at home, only taking six weeks off for the birth of each child.

Though her job was a high priority, so too were her kids, and in order to balance work and spending time with them, Lori and her husband decided to make a financial sacrifice by buying a house a half a block from her office on Capitol Hill so she could go home for lunch and nurse. Avoiding time in the car with the commute to and from work allowed her the time she needed and desired to spend as much of it with her kids, even while juggling her demanding career. Unfortunately, like many parents, she allowed her kids and work to become her highest priorities, forgetting about herself and her own well-being. She admits this was the unhealthiest period of her life.

At the request of Dan Goldin, NASA's ninth and longest tenured Administrator of NASA, Lori began her first tour at NASA in 1996, during the Clinton Administration. It was there that she gained the motivation to run the Marine Corps Marathon. During an early morning staff meeting, overhearing that Lori, along with some of her colleagues, were planning to train for the marathon, a senior official who she knew was not her biggest fan offhandedly blurted out that Lori "could never do that." That was all the motivation she needed to kick-start her workout routine and training, proving to herself and the naysayer that she could do it.

In order to make time for training, Lori came in to the office early every single day for eight straight months, before running the marathon in October 1997. With a daily meeting that started at 7:45 each morning, Lori and two colleagues would arrive at the office by six o'clock, sometimes even earlier for long runs. That was the only time they had if they wanted to train together (and in doing so were able to hold each other accountable) and fit it into their overpacked schedule.

On the weekends, Lori relied on her supportive husband, Dave, to be in charge of the kids so she could get in the required sixteen-, eighteen-, and twenty-mile runs that usually lasted hours and were impossible to accomplish during the workweek. Her husband was great because most times Dave would ride his bike, carrying their three- and five-year-old sons in a back-cart so they could spend time together as they cheered on their mom. Years later when her boys were writing school essays, or filling out their college applications on whom they admired, they would write that they wanted to be as strong and tough as their mom, respecting the fact she got up that early to workout. But none of this—maintaining a schedule and balancing work and family—would have been possible without the help of her partner, Dave, stepping up to the plate. It's important to be with someone who brings out the best in you, allowing you to shift and share priorities together.

## Girl on the Run

My girlfriends poked fun at me a while back and gave me the nickname "girl on the run" because I'm always on the go, moving from place to place and literally running most of the time. Sometimes I was running because I was training for races. Despite the fact that I was visiting new cities while on work travel for my business development gig, I knew that it was imperative that I put in the training time and miles prior to running a big race, especially a marathon.

In this particular case, the race in question was the Marine Corps Marathon in 2015. Halfway through race training, though, my role and responsibilities at work increased, requiring me to travel more, including trips overseas. Knowing I had to keep up with the long runs I was missing out on back at home with my team, I was forced to run alone—all over the world. At first I was nervous that I wouldn't be running fast enough, running without a pacer, but it ended up working out well. On two separate trips to Paris, I ran both the fourteen- and twelve-mile-long runs,

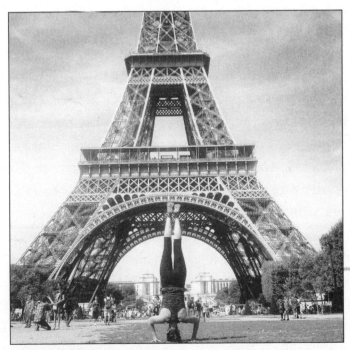

*Laurie A. Watkins enjoying the view of the Eiffel Tower in Paris, France.*

exploring a different part of the city each time, seeing both in completely separate ways. I lost myself in the sounds and sights of each new place. I ran in San Francisco, Maine, New Hampshire, and Virginia. Each adventure allowed me to learn something new about that unfamiliar place and caused me to appreciate my time there even more. By maintaining my running regimen and making the big race a top priority even though there was change and disruption in my work schedule, I allowed myself to train, relieve stress through exercise, keep my sleep schedule, and remain focused through running.

## Find a Work Schedule That Suits Your Family

As a freelance writer, Christine Coppa felt lucky to work from home, though she says it wasn't always that way. She used to be on staff at a magazine where she worked long hours that didn't really match up well with her son JD's daycare pickup. So she took a deep breath and asked her boss if she could work a slightly different schedule where she came in earlier but left in time to get her son from daycare. Her boss was understanding and allowed her to work a more convenient shift. Don't be afraid to express your needs to your employer, or reveal you're a single parent, because most bosses want to work with you, not against you. You can also check out the best companies for working mothers and fathers to target your job search to companies with family-friendly benefits.

When Lori Garver left her NASA policy job in 2001 because a member of a new political party was in charge of the executive branch (George Bush had been elected president), she was suddenly confronted with a unique opportunity.

With Lori's kids now five and seven years old, she realized this was the last opportunity she would have to spend with them while they were young. So she started a consulting firm on her own that allowed her to be home during that period of time. "That five-year-old doesn't remember a time when I wasn't home," she says confidently. From very early on, Lori found creative ways to merge work and family. For her, that was the only way she knew how to sustain balance.

Lori gives a lot of talks on work-life balance for working moms and says she hears people express concern at almost every stage. Many moms subscribe to the worry that when the kids are little and they've had a nanny or are in daycare, they're not going to remember their parents. But Lori argues that that's not going to happen and that parents shouldn't feel guilty about going to work. Children know who their mom or dad is, and in those early years, they don't remember a lot anyway.

Through the eight years that Lori worked at home—years she deemed "the Bush years"—she knew that she eventually wanted to get back to the high-functioning pace and career she led before consulting and shifting focus to her kids. During her time at home, she developed a strategy that included staying active in the space community, so she was able to keep her name fresh in folks' memories. Just as she was leaving NASA, she also was in the process of being elected president of AAS (American Astronautical Society) and served on the Board of Directors for WIA (Women in Aerospace). Lori remained active in these circles even though most of her time was spent in more of a volunteer role. By joining boards and being a member of various organizations, you can use that as a way to remain relevant and active for when you do decide to refocus, changing how you devote your time and with whom you spend it. Lori recommends trying to merge work and family as much as you can. For her, not separating the two was really helpful as she transitioned in and out of various roles in her career.

## True Grit

When he first arrived at West Point, two things really jumped out at Cadet Austin Willard that he wasn't prepared for—the amount of stuff they had cadets do in a day and the amount of time he felt was simply wasted. While the Academy kept him incredibly busy, Austin felt that half the orders assigned were purely a waste of time, not directly contributing to academics. For example, spending time practicing lining up in civil war formations, with WWII era decommissioned rifles, and marching in formation for two-and-a-half hours on a Saturday in order to appear disciplined when there's a parade for a football game seemed unnecessary when Austin would have rather been studying or working on his grad school applications. Notwithstanding the disciplinary aspect of the assignments, Austin didn't feel those things were as important as academics and training. They won't make you a better person in any way, but they certainly eat into your afternoon, he says. Trying to work around that, and trying to stay afloat with the academic course load, is extremely challenging to manage. "I mean I knew it would be busy, but I didn't know how busy," he admits.

On top of Austin's double-majoring in military history and French, he has a fiancée back home in Colorado. When asked how he manages time being a student and keeping in touch, especially living in different time zones, he says, "You have to set clear expectations on the front end with your significant other." Not having time to talk every day or even every week is a reality, but that's the choice Austin made before attending the Academy, and his fiancée has remained true to that. No matter what you're working on, if you don't have someone in your life who is understanding of your priorities and is willing to support them, then it's never going to work. Setting clear expectations is crucial for anyone who is trying to be in a successful long-distance relationship, he says.

One of the toughest decisions Austin had to make after his plebe year was his decision to quit the rugby team. It was tough, because he generally doesn't quit things. Austin loved rugby, he loved the guys, and he loved the sport. But being on the combat weapons team as well and with practice being held three nights a week, usually from right after supper at 6:30 p.m. until 9:30 p.m., then returning to his barracks to start his homework, became unsustainable. For example, Austin's Monday looked like this: wake up at 5 a.m. and lift weights with the rugby team, head to the mess hall and have breakfast, attend classes all day, and then go to rugby practice from 3 p.m. until supper. Most of the time, Austin wouldn't have time to get supper, because he would go straight to the shooting range for combat weapons team practice. He would have somebody bring his supper down, then he would shoot from 6:30 p.m. until 9:30 p.m., get back to his barracks room around 9:30–10 p.m., start his homework, finish his homework around 1 or 2 o'clock in the morning, and then wake up and do it all over again the next morning. That schedule became extremely difficult, and even though his grades didn't suffer, after doing it for one semester, he could just tell that it was not going to be sustainable.

Austin admits that had he kept up with it, he probably could have handled it from a time management perspective if he had an easy major or didn't care about school, but his grades were good enough that he was looking at potentially applying for grad school scholarships like Rhodes, Marshall, etc., and knew that if he let his grades slip at all, that possibility would go away. Plus, having a double major meant that he was already academically overloaded. Then, right after the Christmas break of his second year, he found out he had been accepted to study abroad in France, which meant he would have to be even more overloaded academically before he left, and then again when he came back.

This amazing opportunity forced Austin to be honest with himself and change his priorities a bit. The way he looked at it, he could either do the semester abroad and keep two majors but not play rugby, or he could forego studying abroad, give up a major, and keep playing rugby. And that's really what it came down to. Austin quickly decided he was not going to give up the opportunity to be away from West Point for a semester and get paid to live in France. He also wanted to keep both of his majors and keep his grades up so he could apply for scholarships and get into good grad schools. Realistically evaluating his own time management made the decision easier to let go of rugby, understanding the true meaning of "you can't do everything."

After reading Daniel Pink's book *Drive: The Surprising Truth About What Motivates Us*, Allyson Lewis, founder of

The 7 Minute Life, a time management training and coaching company, learned a little more about the determined men and women of West Point. Pink shared some incredible statistics about the men and women starting at West Point: "Those who are chosen go through six rigorous weeks of cadet basic training—otherwise known as 'Beast Barracks'—before they ever set foot in a classroom. Before the final twelve-mile march that concludes this introductory training, one in twenty of the chosen applicants drops out of the program."

You aren't accepted to West Point unless you're talented and dedicated. But not everyone who is accepted stays. Researchers from West Point, the University of Pennsylvania, and the University of Michigan posed this question: Why is it that some students continued on the road toward military mastery and others got off at the first exit? Their study revealed that those who make the cut and stay the course aren't necessarily stronger or smarter than their peers who quit.

The best predictor of success wasn't intelligence, physical condition, or leadership ability. According to Pink, it was what she defines as "perseverance and passion for long-term goals." Grit is the secret ingredient that empowers us to move from where we are today to where we want to be tomorrow. Grit is the difference between saying, "I'll try to do it" and saying, "I will do it." Grit is critical because repetition— performing the right tasks and thinking the right kinds of things over and over again—strengthens the connections in your brain. Eventually, all that repetition makes it easier to make positive choices and take positive action. Perseverance is what makes that repetition possible. It is this "stick-to-itiveness" that enables you to do what you say you will do and as a result become the person you want to be and live the life you desire.

Perseverance is a choice. It is a commitment to following through on what you say you want to do. It means that:

- If you say you want to be in the best shape of your life, you do what it takes to be in the best shape of your life. You exercise, walk, run, lift weights, do cardio, and make the physical effort to improve your health daily.

- If you say you want to renew and restore your faith, you take daily steps to renew and restore your faith. You read, pray, listen, reach out, and serve the world around you.

- If you say you want to be more competent in your work, you work to become more competent. You study, practice, seek out mentors, and hold yourself accountable to your word.

There are people all around you who are doing what you have said you want to do, living the life you dream of, and accomplishing the goals you set for yourself long ago. You can do the same.

So what's holding you back? Old patterns? Bad habits? If old cognitive models and bad habits are holding you back from achieving your goals, now is the time to create new models and more productive habits. It's time to develop new and stronger neuronal connections that support your desire for a better, more rewarding, and more fulfilling life. Living out your dreams takes work, and sometimes that work feels impossible and fruitless. But when life gets hard, take confidence knowing that it's the tension-filled times of challenge and pressure that produce the deepest levels of growth—and the greatest victories.

While working full-time and training for the 2014 CrossFit Games on the side, Christy Adkins realized that she could potentially train and compete as a professional CrossFit athlete full-time. She was married, her husband Tim was supportive of the idea, and they were both contributing the same amount of income. As a result, Tim couldn't necessarily support both of them, but thanks to Christy's success in CrossFit, she had more and more companies supporting her and her training, which would help supplement their income. Christy felt she could make the leap, and by the middle of 2014, she decided to go very part-time on work and full-time training for the Games.

Realizing that she would not be able to be a professional athlete in the sport without making a full commitment, Christy ultimately decided to quit her job to focus fully on training and competing full-time. Unlike when she decided to become a nurse—which was a long-term career move and one that was going to be a part of her life for many years to come—this new full-time commitment would be for a finite amount of time, similar to a campaign. That mentality made the decision easier because Christy and her husband knew this wasn't a financial decision to set them up for retirement; this was something they knew they could do for a few years because of the support of the companies she had, and it was worth it.

In 2015, after training full-time for that entire year, Christy narrowly missed qualifying for the Games. It was a major blow and affected her self-esteem because she went all in and didn't get what she wanted, missing her goal. She couldn't help but feel like "that's not supposed to happen." After that, she was faced with a choice—to quit, or to keep forging ahead.

Christy had already gone all in for over a year by that point, so she had to ask herself, "Do I keep going and believe in myself knowing I can get even better than I was then?" Perhaps somewhat troublesome was the fact that she had gone into the 2015 Regionals feeling the strongest and best she had ever felt and had ultimately had a good weekend, but she missed her goal. With the support of her husband, coach, and family, she made the decision to go back. After all, if she thought it was a good decision a week ago, why wouldn't it *still* be the right choice for her?

Throughout the year, she made sure to remind herself of that. She needed Tim (her husband) to remind her of that. She also hired a mental coach to help her. Nevertheless, it was a struggle all the time to keep reinforcing the idea of "you are where you need to be, and this is the right path for you right now." Had Christy been alone with her doubts, she could have allowed herself to quit, which is why her support system was so important. As a result, with grit and a strong focus on her time management and training regimen, Christy went on to compete, placing 24th in the world at the 2016 CrossFit Games.

## It's a Marathon, Not a Sprint
During the summer of 2012, the campaign ramped up, and so did the stress. Travel became more common, and the

routine that I had constructed at headquarters felt like it was out the window.

During this time, my biggest battle was against stress. The only way to make it through the 18-hour days, the constant travel, and the unending pressure was to find a way to cope with the stress. For most of my colleagues, that meant going out for drinks at the local alehouses and barrooms, which added more empty calories, late nights, and drunken drama. Since this wasn't my first rodeo (campaign), I was determined to add some sanity to my day. So I took back that "going out" time and made time for myself instead. I made time to make healthy food, time to work out, and time to find my inner peace. I was selective about how I spent that time and with whom I spent it, choosing quality time, like quiet "family dinners" at my house with a core group of supportive coworkers, over a "big night out."

Finding this time for me wasn't easy, but it benefited my sanity and overall well-being. Guarding my own time—and sometimes being a little selfish—was the key to keeping my stress in check during this long, busy stretch of the campaign. It made me a better person, coworker, and friend.

For the last two months of the campaign, I lived on the road, staffing political veterans—people like Mayor Rahm Emanuel and Representative Debbie Wasserman Shultz, who never seemed to need to sleep or eat—who could hit six different events in a day and not break a sweat. With determination, I managed to both eat and sleep while on the road and at home during the insanity of the home stretch of the campaign.

# CHAPTER 8

# THE HOME STRETCH

**Campaign**

(*verb*)

To WORK IN AN ORGANIZED AND ACTIVE WAY TOWARD A
PARTICULAR GOAL.[43]

One of the most surreal parts of any campaign is the day after its expiration date. The office that had been a hive of activity just days before now suddenly has the energy of a deflated balloon. People wander around the war room, cleaning up, removing any trace of a coordinated campaign, and telling stories of days gone by. It is a time when colleagues wake from their caffeine-induced mania of the last few months and try to either get back to their "real" life or figure out their next move. This "Day After" lull can be just as tough on your physical and mental health as the stressful days of the actual campaign. With a sudden lack of structure and purpose, it's easy to slip into a melancholic haze, start eating out of boredom, and lose the inertia to work out.

After working on a dozen or so campaigns throughout my career, I have come to the conclusion that this finite period of time is what motivates some, particularly campaign "lifers" who continue to choose this lifestyle as a career. Unfortunately, a constant campaign environment is not conducive to eating healthy, working out, and getting enough regular sleep.

Over the years I have watched colleagues and friends absolutely torture their bodies by eating junk, gaining weight, and complaining about being tired and feeling like shit, yet they do nothing to change their behavior. Admittedly, I was one of those people back in 2008, and I can honestly say that the way I chose to eat, work out, and sleep during the 2012 presidential campaign, using the tools that were provided to you in this book, proved to be 100 percent beneficial and a drastic improvement from past behavior and campaigns.

## Master Cleanse

It was the summer of 2012, Carly Rae Jepsen's "Call Me Maybe" was stuck in my head, and I saw a big blue box with BluePrint Cleanse splashed across the side being delivered to my colleague Lacey's desk. I walked over and asked, "What is this, please tell me more." I was intrigued and impressed that someone would be doing a cleanse during a reelection campaign. I mean, I was doing a Paleo diet that month myself, but this BluePrint Cleanse appeared to be nothing but juice.

I ordered one for myself and immediately started the following week. Having never done a cleanse before, I did some quick research and realized it was completely doable and would save me a bunch of time that week because I wouldn't need to prepare any meals or cook. I observed my colleague as she went through the week, seeming to be able to hold her shit together. So why couldn't I? "You've got this," I told myself.

After three days, I got over the "empty hole in my stomach" feeling and started to feel completely energized, as if I had given my body a reboot. My skin was clear, my eyes were bright, and I felt like my body was squeaky-clean. I was growing naturally tired a few hours earlier than I normally would, which made falling asleep that much easier when it was time for bed. Overall, I was feeling great. But honestly, I missed food.

On one particular night during the cleanse, I even went out with some colleagues to a wing house to watch Florida State football. It wasn't as bad as I thought it would be, but of course it sucked that I was drinking my dinner while everyone around me threw back a dozen or so buffalo wings. I brought a juice with me for dinner that satisfied me all the way into the fourth quarter, and being out helped keep me away from food and the refrigerator with temptations I would have had if I had been home alone. I made adjustments, changed my priorities that week, and when I went back to my 80/20 Paleo/Whole30 diet, it was a smooth transition, turning it more into a 90/10 balance, not wanting to dirty up my clean body. And for full disclosure, it was not my favorite experience, and one that I have not done since.

## Change That Campaign Mindset

The way the mind of a "campaigner" works is quite fascinating. It's almost as if the mind is somehow tricked into the acceptance of bad habits because it knows there is an end date. It doesn't matter if you're an executive who can't seem to effectively manage your time; or a parent who tells yourself that it's just too much hassle to get the kids up, dressed, and off to the sports club with you in the morning; or the chief of staff who can't seem to power down, even though he knows he needs to get to bed an hour earlier each night instead of continuing to work on that brief. Most campaigners are guilty in some way, shape, or form.

I have come to the conclusion that on a campaign, the most widely uttered start to a sentence is "When the campaign is over, I will. . . ." It's almost as if people think of a campaign as they would a trip to Las Vegas. Except that a campaign lasts for weeks, months, and in some cases years. Along the way, all of the bad habits that you picked up over time eventually turn into an unhealthy lifestyle and unwanted weight gain. As soon as a campaign is over, the weight you gained from all of the greasy pizza, soda, and processed food you happily stuffed into your mouth over the last year comes right along with you—and it doesn't magically fall off on D-Day. It becomes your baggage until you decide to change your lifestyle. What happens on a campaign does not stay on the campaign. Just remember that, so you can remain energized for the next challenge without being afraid of failing before you even get started. With the recommendations and tools shared throughout this book, you are well on your way to making meaningful and lasting changes, resulting in better health and a happier, more well-balanced life.

## Come Out Stronger on the Other Side

As you've gone through your career, have you ever had that moment when you've said to yourself, "Enough is enough"?

This usually comes during a time when the stress is just overwhelming. Perhaps you've been traveling too much, are not enjoying what you are doing professionally, and are in need of a life change, but something seems to be holding you back. You're not alone. I have been through this at least half a dozen times, and only through writing this book was I able to trust myself enough to take that leap, changing my career, focus, and priorities along the way. It can be scary to make major changes in your life while working toward happiness. But all it takes is one small change, which will lead to bigger, better, more impactful, and more rewarding results. Whether you want to lose weight and step up your exercise routine; eliminate chronic pain by changing your lifestyle; go to bed an hour earlier each night, throwing away the sleep aids; feel more relaxed throughout the work day; manage your time more efficiently; or be more present with colleagues and family, you can do any and all of the above if you make the commitment to yourself and follow through.

Elissa Goodman says she does an easy exercise with clients (this usually runs on for weeks), instructing them to get a notebook (or use the notepad on their phone) and write down what they are angry or mad about. It can be a list of ten things, or fifty to a hundred things, but it's important to write them all down, no matter how long the list.

The best time to do this is in the morning, and it's important to continue the exercise until you get to a place where you can release those things on your list. We carry that stuff around with us, according to Elissa. You have to be honest and ask yourself, "What is holding you back from getting what you want?" As you write down all of the things and see them on paper, staring you in the face, you will come to a place where you realize, "Wow, I didn't know I was angry or still mad about that." You need to release it in order to move on, changing other aspects of your life.

Another exercise Elissa has her clients do is write down what they want in their lives. It's important to not just think it, but also to write it down so you can see it and commit to it. It will be as if you're rewiring your brain, telling it, "I want to do this different type of job, or I want to get married, or I want this specific man or woman to come into my life." We need to manifest and visualize the change Elissa recommends. By doing that, it will get you back in touch with your soul and what you really, really want in life. Writing things down is kind of like an old-fashioned way of making things happen. I believe it follows along the same principles as when we make lists to help with time management and achieving our daily tasks. This recommended exercise should motivate you and calm you at the same time while centering you on your goals.

## Are You Present?

With a strong desire to make a change in the way I spend my time with people, and a hope to be more present, with my cell phone out of sight, truly listening and making eye contact, I worked on each and every engagement I had with another person for one whole year. After I read *Presence* by Amy Cuddy, I started cutting out distractions and people in my life that weren't serving me. I found that I had a lot more time than before, and instead of filling that time back up with frivolous things, I spent it with quality people, actively engaged and present. It was not the easiest adjustment to make, but I learned from Cuddy's book that it would be beneficial, not just for those around me, but for myself as well. In the traditional sense, this kind of presence can help you become "more successful," but what matters most is that it will allow you to approach stressful situations without anxiety, fear, and dread and leave them without regret, doubt, and frustration.

As Cuddy acknowledges, change always has the potential to create anxiety within us.

She says that it's all right, though, to have to regain our presence sometimes: "Sometimes we lose it and have to start again, and that's okay."[44]

Presence and empowerment go hand in hand. As Elissa Goodman explains, often her clients don't feel empowered enough to make the hard choices or changes necessary in their life to achieve what they so desperately seek—a happier and healthier life. She hears things like: "I don't have a choice," "I'm stuck in this job," "I'm stuck in this marriage," "I'm stuck in this house," "I'm stuck with this doctor that isn't helping me." The list goes on and on, Elissa says. But she tells each client the same thing: "You have a choice, you're scared, and you are letting fear control you."

Elissa recommends a great book by Louise Hay, *You Can Heal Your Life*, about healing yourself and getting in touch with parts of illnesses that relate to your soul, to different parts of your being and why things are happening. There's always a reason why things are happening around you and why they are the way they are, Hay says. If there are things that don't make you happy or you no longer feel that your job is going well, there's always a reason. And you are usually the one behind that reason. Elissa recommends sitting back and asking yourself, "What am I doing to make this happen or to cause this?" Once you identify the cause, only then can you work to correct, eliminate, or change it. It's crucial that you trust yourself and that you make the right decision.

Continue to remind yourself that you are worth living. Elissa reminds herself every single day that she is worth it in this world and that she is worth having a fantastic life. Elissa wants that for herself, and she also wants to better other people's lives, which is why she became a nutritionist. Through her work, she is able to help other people thrive and be their best self.

## Knowing When to Leave

Even Bill Nye knows what it's like to hit that breaking point, no longer feeling fulfilled in the work he was doing. For him, it happened on October 3, 1986, when he quit his engineering job, having grown tired of working for guys who were just obsessed with making a profit every quarter, and executives making decisions that he disagreed with. That's when Bill decided to be a performer . . . and the rest, of course, is history!

Sometimes, though, it's not the employee's decision when to leave. Almost everyone has been fired at least once in their life, and Bill's first firing came while working in a bike shop at age 15. While growing up in Northwest, Washington, DC, Bill rode his bike 10.1 miles to work each day all the way into Arlington, VA, to a place called Mel Pinto Imports. Mel Pinto was the first to import Gitane bicycles to the U.S., the same bikes ridden by Jacques Anquetil, and it was just cool to be working for the guy. Bill admits he wasn't as big or as strong as a regular bike mechanic and struggled a bit. After just a couple of weeks, his boss said, "Look, you're just not keeping up; you're not strong enough, kid." That was it. He had been fired for not being strong enough or fast enough.

Bill eventually got over it but recommends learning from these kinds of experiences by improving in areas where you're not as strong as you could be, admitting weakness, asking for help, and not feeling defeated. Since we all have room for improvement, take Bill's advice and always remember, "Everyone you will ever meet knows something you don't." By making one small, positive change, you are on your way to a healthier, happier you. We lead busy lives, but we should never be too busy to connect with and make at least one phone call to a parent, sibling, or friend during the day.

## Life is a Balancing Act

As Dan Nevins explains, "The truth is, how I balance it all, is that I don't always balance it all. And the key difference of why it all works for me now is that I am aware that I am unbalanced. Sometimes we get in this routine of actually believing that we're doing everything we can. And most of the time, that's just not true." Dan admits that he knows he can always do more and is aware when things are off. Now that he is self-aware, he works hard to fix the problem, whether that's taking an event off his calendar to avoid overcommitting himself or blocking off weeks at a time to see his children. He makes a point of staying in constant communication and taking the time to touch base every day with his kids and ex-wife.

## Where Do You Get Your Strength?

I asked this question to the following people who shared where they get their strength:

"I get my strength from my inner passion. Knowing I am assisting people with healing themselves (chiropractic, nutrition, self-empowerment) to be greater in the world gives me strength. The love I create for myself also gives me strength, along with my dog, who shows me unconditional love. Hiking in nature shows me that I can do anything, feeling Mother Nature's power." —Dr. Jodi Hodges, Colorado[45]

"I get my strength from my wife, my son, and the people around me. I try and hire people smarter than me, surrounding myself with people that are more ambitious, and that helps drive me." —Jamie Leeds, Washington, DC

"I get my strength from food and enough sleep. Along with that, my parents gave me these ideas:
- We are each responsible for our own actions.
- Leave the world better than you found it.

Those ideas keep me going. When I hear people say something like, 'I was very bad today,' referring to what they chose to eat, I just don't get it. If you admonish yourself for not eating right, just who is taking responsibility for your not eating right—if it's not you?" —Bill Nye, New York

"I get my strength from God and the lessons I've learned through my experiences (both good and bad) . . . from seeing the world through the eyes of innocent and curious children who come through my classroom each year. My passion for motivating children to learn drives me. I get strength from my husband, who supports everything I do and always encourages me to take leaps. Our son, who sees me as his superhero, who can do no wrong. Also from my mother, the epitome of grace, humility, and compassion. From my sisters and their families, who remind me about unconditional love and the 'village' mentality. I can't let these people down, so I always find it in me to keep going, even when it's the hardest thing to do." —Christina Wimberly, Florida[46]

"I get my strength from my connection to God and my family. Taking time for cultivating these connections is essential for me. That means quiet time every day for prayer and meditation, as well as trying to balance work with meaningful time with my family." —Tim Ryan, Ohio[47]

"Having survived greater challenges gives me the confidence, resilience, and tenacity to not back down in the face of resistance. My faith; my husband, who is a true "partner in crime"; my friends; and getting myself to my own "happy place" (rooftop, monastery, chapel, beach, etc.) give me moments to refresh and rebuild amidst the struggles. I've learned to be centered and trust in my own integrity rather than what the world tells me is true." —Rebecca Ballard, Washington, DC.[48]

"I get my strength from the awe of nature. To paraphrase author John Muir, why do we even build churches, if you look around at such places like Yosemite Valley; this is a cathedral that God built that's greater than any that a human could ever build. I was raised a religious person but now [I am] more spiritual in a sense, through the energy of the universe and going outside; being on top of a mountain reminds me that we are all insignificant in the grand picture of things, and to some that may seem scary, as if they don't matter. But to me, it's freeing to realize that if I mess up . . . in the grand scheme of things, it doesn't matter. You will be o.k. It just allows you to do what you need to do and try to make the world a better place. If today isn't a great day, don't worry about it, because in the end, we live in a giant world and eventually we will all turn to dirt." —Jake Frank, Wyoming[49]

"Strength comes in many forms, both seen and unseen. I'd like to think that my strength and drive come from a few key motivating factors: seeking a brighter future, both individually and as a world; competition, again, with oneself and with external forces; and finally, an urge to be a better person to benefit those around me. From playing tug-of-war with one's own past, present, and future self, to trying to be the best player you can be in today's competitive world— motivating factors can sometimes be as thin as the paper this book is written on. But, more importantly, it really lies deep within who we are as humans. An innate sense of self-betterment, togetherness, and seeking a brighter future for our species. I don't know if that's why I get up in the morning, or go for jogs, or try and eat right—or if it's just simply wanting to feel good. But knowing my friends and family are seeking the same answers helps me realize that, most likely, my motivation comes from them." —Phil Larson, Colorado

"My daughters and my wife are my biggest strength. I get a lot of strength when I go to Haiti. I get a lot of strength when I see my team happy each time we open a new restaurant. Hard work, and the moments of hard work, give me strength. It's amazing! Every time you open a new window into the world, you realize how little you know. That's what keeps me going." —José Andrés, Washington, DC

"The backbone of my strength comes from my faith, and the inner drive and passion to be a good steward to myself and others. It comes from my partner, Rob, who brings out the best in me, not the stress in me, forever encouraging me to take chances. Being lost in nature always helps me find myself and see the beauty around me. My grit comes from my passion for living the healthiest, happiest life I can, unafraid to put in the hard work to make it happen. It comes from traveling this spectacular world in search of all that is good, appreciating how other people live and where they come from. And it comes from my dog, Whiskey Bravo, who is my role model for being alive." —Me, Laurie A. Watkins, California

So now, I will ask you the same question that I asked the "Strength Seekers" above.

Where do you get your strength?

Really think about the question before you answer for yourself.

I hope this book has inspired you, motivated you, and empowered you to go out and start making choices toward living the life that you have always dreamed about.

By executing your first "self-nudge," which starts by changing one thing today, you are on the road to making positive, healthier changes to your road map to life. Everything in life is a choice. I hope you choose to become a "Strength Seeker" and command your day, starting now.

# APPENDIX

## Hank's Oyster Stew, by Jamie Leeds[50]
For 4

### Ingredients:

2 large carrots, medium diced

2 large parsnips, medium diced

2 large green zucchini, medium diced

3 shallots, medium diced

1 qt. heavy cream*

2 cup corn

2 cup peas

1 tbsp fresh chopped thyme

24 East Coast Oysters, shucked, reserve liquid

1 cup smoked medium-diced ham

1 cup sea beans

1 tbsp smoked Spanish paprika

Salt and pepper to taste

### Directions:

In a small sauce pan sauté the carrots, parsnips, zucchini, and shallots until tender; add cream and reduce by half. Add the corn, peas, thyme, and reserved oyster liquid. Place 6 oysters in each bowl and pour 4 to 6 oz of the mixture over them. Top with 7 to 8 pieces of ham, a few sea beans, and a sprinkle of paprika for garnish.

*If you are looking for a low-fat or vegetarian heavy cream substitute, try blending tofu with unflavored soy milk until the mixture is smooth. This substitute is a healthy alternative for heavy cream.

## Paleo Phil's Meatballs and Arrabiata Sauce (optional)[51]
Serves: Makes about 15 to 20 meatballs

### Ingredients:

⅔ lb grass-fed ground beef

⅔ lb ground Italian sausage

⅔ lb ground turkey

1 tsp crushed red pepper flakes

1 large organic egg

1 tsp sea salt

¾ tsp black pepper

1 tbsp olive oil

1 half diced organic sweet onion

4 cloves minced of organic garlic

½ bag of fresh organic riced cauliflower (Trader Joe's)

## Directions:

Preheat your oven to 400 degrees F. Line a baking sheet with foil or parchment paper. Combine the ingredients—beef, sausage, turkey, pepper flakes, egg, salt, and pepper in a large bowl, and mix with clean hands to combine. Sauté the diced onion, minced garlic, and riced cauliflower in 1 tbsp of olive oil on medium heat until onion is translucent and cauliflower is soft. Set aside for a few moments to cool and then fold the onion, garlic, and cauliflower into the mixture in the bowl. Gently roll the meat into golf-size balls and place on the baking sheet. Repeat this with remaining meat. Bake for about 14 to 18 minutes or until meat is cooked all the way through. Serve with Phil's Arrabiata Sauce.

Note: These freeze well. To thaw, simmer them in broth or pasta sauce until they've softened.

## Paleo Phil's Arrabiata Sauce
Serves: 4

## Ingredients:

2 (28 oz) cans of organic diced tomatoes

2 tbsp light olive oil

4 cloves of organic minced garlic

⅔ tsp sea salt and pepper

⅓ cup chopped fresh basil

1 tsp crushed red pepper flakes

## Directions:

In large saucepan, combine tomatoes and olive oil. Simmer for 20 to 25 minutes. Stir in garlic, salt, and pepper, and let simmer an additional 10 minutes. Remove from heat and mix in basil and red pepper flakes.

## Elissa's Breakfast Boosting Acai Bowl and Granola[52]
Serves: 2

### Ingredients:

4-pack of Açai berry puree

2 cups almond milk (or water)

2 bananas

1 cup frozen strawberries

2 tbsp hemp protein powder

Fresh berries

4 tbsp hemp seeds

### Directions:

Combine all ingredients in a blender until smooth. Top with granola (recipe below), fresh berries, and hemp seeds.

## Elissa's Heart-Healthy Granola
Yields: 7 cups

### Ingredients:

3 cups organic old-fashioned gluten-free oats

1 cup raw, sprouted nuts and seeds (walnuts, almonds, sunflower seeds)

⅛ cup organic coconut sugar

¼ cup organic unsulphured shredded coconut

½ tsp organic cinnamon

½ tsp Himalayan pink sea salt

⅙ cup organic maple syrup

½ tsp organic pure vanilla extract

1 ½ tbsp organic coconut oil or grapeseed oil

### Directions:

Preheat oven to 325 degrees F. Mix all dry ingredients in a big bowl. Pour maple syrup, vanilla extract, and oil over the ingredients and mix to coat evenly. Spread the mixture onto an ungreased baking sheet. Put in the oven for 35 minutes, checking often. Remove from the oven and let cool completely.

Note: To make a crunchier, clumpier granola, you can add two beaten egg whites to the wet mixture.

## Elissa's Chocolate Chip Protein Bars
Makes 12 bars

### Ingredients:

1 ½ cups raw, sprouted cashews

sea salt

10 to 12 pitted organic Medjool dates

4 tbsp organic shredded coconut

2 tsp organic vanilla extract

¼ cup nondairy/vegan dark chocolate chips

¼ cup organic hemp seeds

### Directions:

Put cashews into food processor with pinch of salt and process until crumbled. Add the dates and process until well combined. Add coconut, vanilla extract, chocolate chips, and hemp seeds and pulse until combined into sticky dough. Line an 8×8 pan with parchment paper, hanging over the edges. Place mixture into pan and flatten with your hand or a spatula. Freeze for 20 to 30 minutes. Remove from freezer and pull out of pan by lifting the parchment paper. Cut into 12 bars. Store in an airtight container in the fridge. For easy travelling, tightly wrap the individual bars. If you're looking for an extra boost of antioxidants or another healthy grab-and-go item that you can put in a jar and store in the fridge, you've got to make Elissa's Chia Pudding. Eating a small amount of this low-calorie food will help brighten your skin, fight off signs of aging, and protect you from disease. Plus, chia seeds also have three times the amount of fiber in oatmeal, two times the amount of protein in any other bean, seed, or grain, and two times the amount of potassium in a banana.

## Elissa's Chia Breakfast Pudding

½ cup unsweetened organic almond milk

2 tbsp chia seeds

2 tbsp organic sulphite-free raisins

generous sprinkle of organic cinnamon

1 dried chopped organic date, pit removed

½ tsp alcohol-free vanilla

dried stevia herb powder

1 organic avocado

2 tbsp more almond milk for blending

### Directions:

Combine ½ cup almond milk, chia, raisins, cinnamon, chopped date, and vanilla and let stand for 5 to 10 minutes until it thickens. Blend the mixture with the dried stevia powder and avocado, adding almond milk for consistency. Test to see if chia seeds are smooth. If you own a really powerful blender, the chia seeds should totally disappear.

---

### Elissa's Seed Facts:
#### Choose Chia for High Fiber

Chia seeds contain 11 grams of dietary fiber per ounce, about half of the daily recommended amount for women (and one-third the amount for men). Adding chia into your diet can help you to balance blood sugar levels, lower cholesterol, improve digestion, and aid in weight loss. Flaxseeds are also a great option, with 8 grams per ounce.

### Up Your Omega-3s with Flaxseed

Flaxseeds contain 6.4 grams per one ounce serving size. They provide alpha-linolenic acid (ALA), the type of omegas found in plant-based sources. You still need sources of EPA and DHA fatty acids, found in fish. If you're not a fan of whole flax, consider ground flaxseed, which blends seamlessly into smoothies and baking goods.

### Hemp Provides a Plant-Based Protein Boost

Hemp seeds are the clear protein provider. They contain 9 grams of plant-based, complete protein per ounce, making them the perfect addition to postworkout smoothies. Make homemade granola bars and add a scoop, sprinkle over coconut yogurt with fruit, and even add to salads to protein-boost your lunch.

### Tips for Storage

Seeds contain oils that can spoil them quickly. Therefore, I always recommend that you store seeds in the refrigerator. Keep them in airtight containers, like a mason jar, to prevent oxidation. It can be tempting to buy in bulk, but be sure to label with the expiration date and tape onto your storage container.

Alternatively, you can store in the freezer for a longer shelf life.

### How to Consume

- Flaxseeds are best freshly ground; you can purchase whole, then add to your coffee grinder and grind "to order." After this, add to smoothies, into your recipes for homemade oat or granola bars, into baked good recipes, or use as "breadcrumb" coating or as an egg substitute (2 tablespoons water mixed with 2 tablespoons ground flax=1 egg).

- Chia seeds can easily be used to make chia pudding, or chia jam. Add a tablespoon to your lemon water, allow to sit for 2 to 3 minutes, then stir and enjoy. Or add into your yogurt with fresh fruit, blend into smoothies, and add into juices.
- Hemp seeds make a great addition to soups and salads; you can puree into soups for a "creamy" texture, add to granola, use as a garnish for your yogurt, or add into smoothies.

## Elissa's Matcha Green Tea Latte
Serving Size: 1

### Ingredients:

½ cup organic Unsweetened Almond Milk

½ cup organic So Delicious Culinary Coconut Milk

½ to 1 tsp organic Ceremonial DōMatcha Tea

7 to 10 drops 100% pure Omica vanilla stevia (adjust depending on your desired sweetness)

1 tsp pure vanilla powder

½ tsp cinnamon

1 tbsp organic coconut oil or Bulletproof XCT Oil

1 tbsp grass-fed butter or ghee

### Directions:

Add all ingredients to blender/Vitamix. Blend until smooth and creamy. Heat on stovetop or in the microwave.

## Laurie's Good Juice

### Ingredients:

2 long stalks of celery

1 sprig of mint

1 medium size red/gold beet (+ 2 leaves from beet)

½ slice of lemon

1 inch of ginger root

1 to 2 stems of parsley and leaves

1 regular size carrot

1 small green apple

1 leaf of green chard

### Directions:

Run all ingredients through a standard juicer at regular speed. Drink within 12 hours and cover any stored excess juice.

## Elissa's Marinated Tempeh

### Ingredients:

2 tbsp Bragg's apple cider vinegar

2 tbsp organic coconut aminos

1 tsp organic sesame oil

1 tsp grated ginger

juice of one lime

8 oz. organic tempeh, cut into thin strips

1 tbsp coconut oil

### Directions:

Prepare the tempeh marinade by whisking together the vinegar, coconut aminos, sesame oil, ginger, and lime. Place cut thin tempeh strips in a small dish and pour the marinade over, being sure each piece is covered in the marinade. Marinate for a minimum of 2 hours.

Heat the coconut oil over medium high heat in a large sauté pan. Cook each side of tempeh until browned, approx. 3 to 4 minutes on each side. Set cooked tempeh aside and complete salad.

## Elissa's Detox Dressing*

### Ingredients and Directions:

In a food processer, combine:

handful of parsley

handful of cilantro

handful of basil

garlic clove

sea salt

1 tbsp olive oil

*Use on salads, veggies, eggs, omelets, and over various protein. Cilantro and parsley are beneficial because they bind to heavy metal toxins, pulling them out of the body.

## Elissa's Hummus

### Ingredients:

4 cups organic garbanzo beans, drained

¼ cup organic tahini paste

¼ cup organic lemon juice

1 tsp organic ground cumin

⅓ cup organic extra virgin olive oil

1 tsp organic chopped jalapeño chile

½ bunch stemmed organic cilantro

1 tsp organic chopped garlic

¾ tbsp organic raw honey

¾ tbsp Himalayan pink sea salt

### Directions:

Combine all ingredients in a food processor and blend until smooth. Adjust seasonings to taste.

## Laurie's Crock-Pot Chicken Enchilada Stew

Serves: 4 to 6

### Ingredients:

2 lbs chicken breasts

1 chopped green bell pepper

1 (4 oz) can chopped jalapenos

1 (4 oz) can chopped green chiles

1 chopped yellow onion

2 tbsp coconut oil

1 (14 oz) can diced tomatoes

1 (7 oz) can tomato sauce

3 minced garlic cloves

1 tbsp cumin

1 ½ tbsp chili powder

2 ½ tsp dried oregano

salt and pepper, to taste

bundle of cilantro, to garnish

avocado, place on top with cilantro garnish

### Directions:

Start with a medium to large size Crock-Pot, add your chicken breasts. Then add the rest of the ingredients on top of the chicken, in any order. Turn the knob of your Crock-Pot to the low setting for 8 to 10 hours or the high setting for 6 to 8 hours. After the chicken is done cooking and has marinated in the ingredients and its own juices, use tongs or two forks to pick at the chicken and shred it while mixing in with all of the ingredients, creating a delicious stew. Dish yourself a few scoops of chicken (including the juice in the pot) in a bowl. Top with cilantro and some avocado slices.

## Elissa's Summer Vegetable Minestrone
Serves: 6

### Ingredients:

2 tbsp organic coconut oil

1 small diced white onion

1 small thinly sliced leek

1 large diced heirloom carrot

2 chopped celery stalks

¼ cup finely chopped fresh herbs (rosemary, thyme, oregano, and sage)

2 diced garlic cloves

Salt and pepper to taste

1 ear organic corn, cut off the cob

¼ lb white asparagus, cut into 1-inch chunks

¼ lb diced artichoke hearts (fresh or frozen)

½ cup green beans, cut into 1-inch chunks

⅓ cup uncooked English peas

¼ lb thinly sliced mushrooms, (your choice of edible mushrooms; Elissa uses brown buttons)

2 whole bay leaves

14-ounce container of finely diced tomatoes (Elissa uses Pomo)

3 cups organic vegetable or chicken stock

1 cup organic kidney beans

3 cups spinach (could also use kale, watercress, or collard greens)

### Directions:

Heat the coconut oil in a 6-quart pot over medium heat. Add the onion, leek, carrots, celery, and fresh herbs and sauté for 3 to 5 minutes. Add the garlic and sauté a few more minutes, while stirring occasionally. Season with salt and pepper. Add in the corn, asparagus, artichoke, green beans, peas, mushrooms, and bay leaves. Continue to sauté for another 5 minutes. Add the tomatoes, stock, and kidney beans and allow to simmer on low for 10 minutes, stirring occasionally. Add the spinach (or greens of your choice) last and finish with a final 5-minute simmer. Remove the bay leaves, which should have floated to the top and season with additional salt and pepper if needed. Can also be served with gluten-free quinoa pasta shells.

## Laurie's Paleo/Whole30 Panang Chicken Curry with Cauliflower Rice
Serves: 4

### Ingredients:

1 tbsp coconut oil

2 tbsp Panang curry paste

1 14.5 oz can of organic coconut milk

1 organic thinly sliced small onion

5 organic leaves of Thai basil

1 ½ lbs organic boneless skinless chicken breast cut into 1-inch pieces

1 thinly sliced organic red bell pepper

½ head of organic broccoli, cut into florets

1 tsp Red Boat fish sauce

4 cups cooked cauliflower rice (see recipe below) or 1 whole organic cauliflower head

### Directions:

Melt the coconut oil in a large pan over medium heat. Add the curry paste and sauté for 2 minutes until fragrant. Add half of the can of coconut milk and stir, cooking for an additional 3 minutes. Add the remaining coconut milk, onion, and Thai basil. Bring to a boil and then reduce heat to a simmer for 5 minutes. Add the chicken breast pieces, bell pepper, broccoli, and fish sauce. Simmer for 6 to 8 minutes until the chicken is cooked through, stirring often. Remove pan from heat and remove chicken from pan, placing in separate bowl. Shred chicken into small- to medium-sized pieces. Throw shredded chicken back into pan, soaking up curry sauce and mixing with the vegetables. Plate your meal by placing curry on top of cauliflower rice, garnished with parsley (optional).

## Cauliflower rice

Chop cauliflower head into florets, size suitable for your processor. In a food processor, chop the florets until they appear small enough, the size of rice. Sauté cauliflower rice in 1 tbsp coconut oil in pan on medium heat, covering for 5 to 7 minutes so rice gets tender. Remove from pan and empty into bowl, fluffing rice with fork.

## Laurie's Light and Spicy Baked Coconut Fish
Serves: 2

### Ingredients:

2 tbsp coconut oil
2 egg whites
1 tbsp almond flour
½ tbsp garlic powder
¼ tbsp baking powder

1 cup unsweetened coconut
  flakes
1 tsp red pepper flakes
1-2 fillets of white fish

### Directions:

Lightly grease a glass pan with coconut oil and set off to the side. Beat egg whites in a bowl. In a separate bowl, combine flour, garlic powder, baking powder, coconut flakes, and red pepper. Coat fillet in egg white mixture and then coat in flour/coconut mix and place on greased pan and bake for 40 minutes at 350 degrees F. Remove from oven and enjoy.

## Laurie's Paleo/Whole30 Slow-Roasted Pork Tenderloin with Dry Rub
Serves: 4

### Dry Rub Ingredients:

(for 2 to 3 lbs of pork roast)
1 ½ tbsp paprika
1 tsp garlic powder

1 tsp dry mustard
1 ½ tsp coarse sea salt

1 (2 to 3 lbs of pork roast,
  preferably shoulder or Boston

butt. Rinse and pat dry with
paper towel, and set aside)

**Dry Rub Directions:**

Mix the paprika, garlic powder, dry mustard, and sea salt together in a small bowl. Rub the spice blend all over the pork. Cover and refrigerate for at least 1 hour, or up to overnight.

**Pork Tenderloin Directions:**

Preheat the oven to 300 degrees F. Stick an instant-read thermometer into the thickest part of the pork, which should register 170 degrees, but basically you want to roast the meat until it's falling apart. Put the pork in a roasting pan and roast for about five hours (for a 2-to-3-lb cut of meat). Use a fork to pull apart the delicious meat, which will be crispy on the outside. The best part!

Transfer the pulled pork tenderloin to a saucepan (include all the crispy bits and pieces) and on low heat, pour ½ cup BBQ sauce on top of meat. Do not stir the meat and sauce together this will mess with the natural moisture and juice of the meat. Instead, make sure the meat is covered with the sauce, cover with a lid, and heat on low heat for twenty minutes. Remove lid, gently stir meat and sauce together, and serve.

If you're looking for a fantastic, premade Paleo/Whole30 approved BBQ Sauce, I recommend Tessemae's Matty's BBQ Sauce. If you can't find it, or want to make your own sauce, here is a basic Paleo BBQ recipe.

### Laurie's Easy Peasy Paleo BBQ Sauce
Serving Size: 1 ½ cups

**Ingredients:**

15 oz. organic tomato sauce
1 cup water

½ cup apple cider vinegar
⅓ cup honey

1 tbsp lemon juice

2 tsp onion powder

1 ½ tsp ground black pepper

1 ½ tsp ground mustard

1 tsp paprika

## Directions:

Combine all of the ingredients in a medium saucepan over medium-high heat. Stir to combine. Bring to a boil, and then reduce to simmer for 1 hour. Taste and adjust seasonings as desired. Serve with meat or store in an airtight container in the refrigerator.

## Laurie's Things in the Fridge Frittata

Serves: 4

I call this the "Things in the Fridge Frittata" because I literally created it using ingredients I found in the fridge. I highly recommend you use a good pan, avocado/coconut oil spray (to generously coat bottom and sides), and fresh eggs (within a week of purchase).

## Ingredients:

10 eggs

1 sprig of rosemary

Chopped pepper (the sweeter the better, don't overdo it, only need about 20 small chunks)

2 to 3 strips of uncured, organic bacon, already cooked and chopped

1 small piece of smoked Gouda chopped into about 10 to 15 mini-pieces

3 sprigs chopped parsley

2 pieces of gluten-free bread (your choice)

## Directions:

Preheat oven to 425 degrees F. Whisk 10 eggs together in a bowl and set aside. Spray bottom and sides of pan with oil. Pull apart pieces of bread and line bottom of pan. Add all chopped meat and veggies to egg mixture and stir well. Drizzle egg mixture all over bread-lined pan, evenly distributing mixture until it reaches the edge of the pan. Bake in the oven for 15 minutes at 425 degrees F, or until cheese is bubbling. Turn the broiler on high for 4 min. to brown the top (if desired) and remove from oven. Remember to be mindful of the HOT handle. Let cool for 2 to 3 few minutes before cutting into slices. Serve with a side of fruit and avocado.

## Laurie's Whole30 Roasted Potatoes and Apples w/ Fresh Rosemary and Himalayan Salt
Serves: 4

### Ingredients:

2 large white potatoes

2 small apples (yellow or green work best)

1 tsp extra virgin olive oil (evoo)

1 tbsp fresh rosemary

Salt, to taste

### Directions:

Heat oven to 350 degrees F. Cut up potatoes and apples into small wedges and throw into a mixing bowl. Drizzle or brush with evoo, sprinkle with rosemary leaves and salt, then mix together contents with your hands. Gently pour contents in bowl out on tin-foil-covered pan, making sure it's spread evenly, and roast for 45 minutes. Halfway through cook time, flip potatoes on pan to get a nice crispy outside. For the last 5 min. of cooking, I like to set the oven on broil and cook on high heat until crispy. Remove from pan and serve hot and crispy.

# ACKNOWLEDGMENTS

I would like to express my gratitude to the many people who saw me through this book, and to all those who provided support, talked things over, read, wrote, offered comments, allowed me to quote their remarks, and assisted in the editing, proofreading, and design.

I would like to thank God for his strength, wisdom, and direction. It was you who helped point me in the right direction. President Obama and Mrs. Obama, thank you for giving me hope and the belief that I can make change. You have both done remarkable things for our country, making it stronger because of your renewed sense of purpose and optimism. You afforded me the opportunity to experience the highest honor of my life, and I am forever grateful. Thank you.

A huge thank-you to Skyhorse Publishing for enabling me to publish this book, and to Julie Ganz, my editor who gave me a long leash, fully supporting me along the way. To Maryann Karinch, my teacher, my voice of reason, and my agent. I am so grateful that the universe brought us together and that I have you watching my back. To Chelsey Marie, thank you for redesigning my life. Tara Zirker, you are a breath of fresh air. Thank you for your light and wisdom. Meg Biram, thank you for sharing your world of creativity and collaboration.

Thank you to all of the Office "Bullies" for being difficult, incorrigible, pains in the ass. For years, you've gone out of your way by putting up roadblocks, creating challenges, and acting malicious toward anyone you feel threatened by in the workplace. Here's a little secret I'll share with you—everyone in the office knows what you're up to. The jig is up. When you treat people with disrespect, belittle your subordinates, or hold someone back due to your own insecurities and inadequacies, you are not only hurting them, but your entire organization. Don't be a bully. While a boss gives orders to his/her employees, a leader influences his/her followers by setting an example. Lift up your team by providing passion, insight, honesty, and a healthy working environment.

CrossFit MPH, CrossFit 813, CrossFit Praxis, and CrossFit Pick Axe, thank you for teaching me to have self-confidence with my body, proper technique, and the true meaning of inner strength. It turns out that being strong is, in fact, beautiful. Thanks for proving me wrong. Danielle Dionne, thank you for your constant motivation and for what you do everyday by turning working professionals into athletes. To Nicole and Ashley Watkins, please never allow anyone or anything to come between your ultimate health and happiness—even yourself. You are both incredibly strong.

Bill Nye, thank you for being a brilliant mentor and friend. Over the years you have pushed me to do more, challenged me to be better, and provided me with more wisdom than I deserve.

Melissa Hartwig, my first Whole30 was life-changing. Thank you for creating a program that changed my relationship with food and created lifelong, healthy habits.

Andrea Hirsekorn, my best mate. Throughout this entire process you supported me, listened to me, and took my phone calls in the middle of the night. Thank you. Jenna Vandenberg, thank you for your help in getting me heard, even in the nosiest of spaces. Matthew Kaplan, thank you for the invitations, yoga, and words of encouragement. You never stopped bringing me inspiration. Thanks, Kap.

Max Holtzman, thank you for never laughing at my wild ideas and for always asking how you could help. Alao Hogan, your motivation turned into healthy competition for me when I needed it most. Your drive, determination, and passion helped remind me that it is never acceptable to accept the status quo. Nan Rich, you will always be my first boss and the woman who taught me how to be a professional, and a lady. Thank you for teaching me compassion, truth, and grace.

Alain Jean, my twin, best friend. What can I say? You were the biggest motivator for me to write this book. You always make me think *BIG*, Alain. What a life! Teddy Johnston, thank you for your friendship, encouragement, and for always knowing who to call. Heidi Nel, thank you for your support and belief in my mission to bring health, happiness, and well-being to the hustlers of the world. Francisco Sanchez, thank you for your help and support throughout the years. Frank Aum, thanks for getting me in the door. It was your invitation that helped me find my strength.

Greg Bowman, thank you for your unwavering support and mentorship throughout my career. You have helped open so many doors for me, and I only hope to be able to return the favor someday. Daniel Serrano, the "locomotive." You make sure every train runs on time and that everyone is taken care of. You are sharp and wise beyond your years. Muchas gracias. Alice McKeon, you helped get this whole thing off the ground when I came to you with not much more than an idea and a file full of unorganized stories. You helped give me wings. Auntie Julie, thank you for your patience, love, and for letting me escape to the Maine woods whenever I got the itch. I admire you for being the strongest woman I know, and you were given this life because you're strong enough to live it.

Stephanie Young, somehow we were able to save each other from the campaign, and ourselves. I will never forget our late-night talks on the couch, family dinners, and bimonthly strategy sessions from our top-secret, off-campus location. You never let me lose faith. Steve Schale, "Thanks, coach." Thank you to my parents and brother, John, for your constant motivation to make you proud. At times it's been hard to live up to, but it only made me stronger. Kristin Carter, I want to thank you for choosing my name out of the pile of résumés when you selected *me* as your intern back in 2003. You broke me in, introducing me to the exciting world of government and politics. Thanks a lot (wink, wink).

And finally, Robert Hess, thank you for your trust, support, faith, and commitment to *our* plan. You are sharp, funny, strong, and insightful. Your presence makes my life and our world so much better. Without you, this would still be a dream, and because of you I am living my dream. I love you.

# ENDNOTES

1. Amy Cuddy, *Presence* (Little, Brown & Company, 2015), p. 142–143.
2. Charles Duhigg, *The Power of Habit: Why We Do What We Do in Life and Business* (Random House, 2014), p. 7.
3. William James, *The Stream of Consciousness* (Psychology, 1892), Chapter 8: The Laws of Habit.
4. Charles Duhigg, *The Power of Habit: Why We Do What We Do in Life and Business* (Random House, 2014), p. 7.
5. Shonda Rhimes interviewed by Oprah Winfrey on Super Soul Sunday, OWN Network, November 15, 2015; http://www.supersoul.tv/supersoul-sunday/full-episode-shonda-rhimes/.
6. Amy Cuddy, *Presence* (Little, Brown & Company, 2015), extracts from p. 253–257.
7. Interview with Stacey Colino on "Secrets to Setting and Maintaining A Routine," October 21, 2015, Washington, DC.
8. Cedric X. Bryant, PhD, Chief Science Officer, American Council on Exercise, December 9, 2015, Seattle, WA.

9. Interview with Stacey Colino on "Secrets to Setting and Maintaining A Routine," October 21, 2015, Washington, DC.

10. Ibid.

11. Ibid.

12. Congressman Tim Ryan, U.S. House of Representatives, November, 23, 2015, Washington, DC.

13. Interview with Stacey Colino on "Secrets to Setting and Maintaining A Routine," October 21, 2015, Washington, DC.

14. Ibid.

15. In-person interview with José Andrés, June 21, 2016, Washington, DC.

16. http://beefsteakveggies.com/who-we-are/.

17. In-person interview with Jamie Leeds, May 26, 2016, in Washington, DC.

18. In-person interview with Lori Garver, July 5, 2016, in Washington, DC.

19. Interview with Phil Larson via Skype, April 20, 2016, Washington, DC via Los Angeles, CA.

20. Interview via FaceTime with Christy Adkins, May 24, 2016, in Washington, DC.

21. Ibid.

22. In-person interview with Bill Nye, May 1, 2016, in Washington, DC.

23. Liza Barnes and Nicole Nichols, "The Benefits of Growing Your Own Food." http://www.sparkpeople.com/resource/nutrition_articles.asp?id=1275&page=2 .

24. Marisa Moore, "Kids in the Garden: Nutritious and Fun." http://www.eatright.org/resource/food/

nutrition/eating-as-a-family/kids-in-the-garden-nutritious-and-fun.

25. Interview via Skype with Austin Willard, May 31, 2016, in Washington, DC.

26. Interview via FaceTime with Elissa Goodman, July 21, 2016, in Washington, DC.

27. "Sleep Health Index 2014." National Sleep Foundation. https://sleepfoundation.org/sleep-health-index.

28. "ACP Recommends Cognitive Behavioral Therapy as Initial Treatment for Chronic Insomnia." American College of Physicians. https://www.acponline.org/acp-newsroom/acp-recommends-cognitive-behavioral-therapy-as-initial-treatment-for-chronic-insomnia.

29. Interview via phone with Dr. Ron Kotler, June 2, 2016, from Lovell, Maine, to Philadelphia, PA.

30. Interview via FaceTime with Elissa Goodman, July 21, 2016, in Washington, DC.

31. "Physical Activity Impacts Overall Quality of Sleep." National Sleep Foundation. https://sleepfoundation.org/sleep-news/study-physical-activity-impacts-overall-quality-sleep.

32. "ACP Recommends Cognitive Behavioral Therapy as Initial Treatment for Chronic Insomnia." American College of Physicians. https://www.acponline.org/acp-newsroom/acp-recommends-cognitive-behavioral-therapy-as-initial-treatment-for-chronic-insomnia.

33. "Circadian rhythm." *ScienceDaily*. https://www.sciencedaily.com/terms/circadian_rhythm.htm.

34. Oprah Winfrey, "What Oprah Knows for Sure About Finding the Fullest Expression of Yourself." *O, The*

*Oprah Magazine*. February 2012. http://www.oprah. com/health/oprah-on-stillness-and-meditation- oprah-visits-fairfield-iowa/all#ixzz4IZQnlyfS.

35. In-person interview with Staff Sgt. Dan Nevins, U.S. Army (medically retired), May 11, 2016, in Washington, DC.

36. "Employer-Reported Workplace Injury and Illness Summary." United States Department of Labor. October 27, 2016. https://www.bls.gov/news.release/ osh.nr0.htm.

37. "Stress management." Mayo Clinic. April 21, 2016. http://www.mayoclinic.org/healthy-lifestyle/stress- management/in-depth/stress-relief/art-20044456?pg=2.

38. Ibid.

39. Interview via with Jake Frank, via FaceTime, September 3, 2016, at Glacier National Park.

40. Florence Williams, "This is your Brain on Nature." *National Geographic*. January 2016. http://ngm. nationalgeographic.com/2016/01/call-to-wild-text.

41. Frankki Bevins and Aaron De Smet, "Making time management the organization's priority." *McKinsley Quarterly*. January 2013. http://www.mckinsey. com/business-functions/organization/our-insights/ making-time-management-the-organizations- priority.

42. Peter Bregman, "A personal approach to organizational time management." *McKinsley Quarterly*. January 2013. http://www.mckinsey.com/business-functions/ organization/our-insights/a-personal-approach-to- organizational-time-management.

43. *Oxford Dictionaries.* Oxford University Press. https://en.oxforddictionaries.com/definition/campaign.

44. Amy Cuddy, *Presence* (Little, Brown & Company, 2015), extracts from pages 25–26.

45. Quote provided by Dr. Jodi Hodges via email, September 7, 2016.

46. Quote provided by Christina Wimberley via email, September 7, 2016.

47. Quote provided by Tim Ryan via email, August, 29 2016.

48. Quote provided by Rebecca Ballard via email, September 7, 2016.

49. Interview with Jake Frank, via Skype, September 3, 2016, in Washington, DC.

50. From Jamie Leeds. Reprinted with permission.

51. From Phil Larson. Reprinted with permission.

52. From Elissa Goodman. https://elissagoodman.com. Reprinted with permission.